Pediatric Orthopedics

Editor

P. CHRISTOPHER COOK

PEDIATRIC CLINICS
OF NORTH AMERICA

www.pediatric.theclinics.com

Consulting Editor
BONITA F. STANTON

December 2014 • Volume 61 • Number 6

ELSEVIER

1600 John F. Kennedy Boulevard • Suite 1800 • Philadelphia, Pennsylvania, 19103-2899

http://www.theclinics.com

THE PEDIATRIC CLINICS OF NORTH AMERICA Volume 61, Number 6
December 2014 ISSN 0031-3955, ISBN-13: 978-0-323-32670-4

Editor: Kerry Holland
Developmental Editor: Casey Jackson

The Pediatric Clinics of North America (ISSN 0031-3955) is published bimonthly by Elsevier Inc., 360 Park Avenue South, New York, NY 10010-1710. Months of issue are February, April, June, August, October, and December. Periodicals postage paid at New York, NY and additional mailing offices. Subscription prices are $200.00 per year (US individuals), $493.00 per year (US institutions), $270.00 per year (Canadian individuals), $657.00 per year (Canadian institutions), $325.00 per year (international individuals), $657.00 per year (international institutions), $100.00 per year (US students and residents), and $165.00 per year (international and Canadian residents and students). To receive students/resident rare, orders must be accompanied by name of affiliated institution, date of term, and the signature of program/residency coordinator on institution letterhead. Orders will be billed at individual rate until proof of status is received. Foreign air speed delivery is included in all Clinics subscription prices. All prices are subject to change without notice. **POSTMASTER:** Send address changes to The Pediatric Clinics of North America, Elsevier Health Sciences Division, Subscription Customer Service, 3251 Riverport Lane, Maryland Heights, MO 63043. **Customer Service: 1-800-654-2452 (US and Canada). From outside of the US and Canada: 1-314-447-8871. Fax: 1-314-447-8029. For print support, E-mail: JournalsCustomerService-usa@elsevier.com. For online support, E-mail: JournalsOnlineSupport-usa@elsevier.com.**

Reprints. For copies of 100 or more, of articles in this publication, please contact the Commercial Reprints Department, Elsevier Inc., 360 Park Avenue South, New York, NY 10010-1710. Tel.: 212-633-3874; Fax: 212-633-3820; E-mail: reprints@elsevier.com.

The Pediatric Clinics of North America is also published in Spanish by McGraw-Hill Inter-americana Editores S.A., Mexico City, Mexico; in Portuguese by Riechmann and Affonso Editores, Rua Comandante Coelho 1085, CEP 21250, Rio de Janeiro, Brazil; and in Greek by Althayia SA, Athens, Greece.

The Pediatric Clinics of North America is covered in MEDLINE/PubMed (Index Medicus), Excerpta Medica, Current Contents, Current Contents/Clinical Medicine, Science Citation Index, ASCA, ISI/BIOMED, and BIOSIS.

PROGRAM OBJECTIVE
The goal of the *Pediatric Clinics of North America* is to keep practicing physicians and residents up to date with current clinical practice in pediatrics by providing timely articles reviewing the state-of-the-art in patient care.

TARGET AUDIENCE
All practicing pediatricians, physicians and healthcare professionals who provide patient care to pediatric patients.

LEARNING OBJECTIVES
Upon completion of this activity, participants will be able to:
1. Review the assessment and treatment of pediatric and adolescent knee, foot, and hip pain.
2. Discuss the evaluation and treatment of scoliosis in the pediatric patient.
3. Describe the evaluation and treatment of slipped capital femoral epiphysis in the pediatric patient and the evaluation and treatment of hip dysplasia in the newborn and infant patient.

ACCREDITATION
The Elsevier Office of Continuing Medical Education (EOCME) is accredited by the Accreditation Council for Continuing Medical Education (ACCME) to provide continuing medical education for physicians.

The EOCME designates this enduring material for a maximum of 15 *AMA PRA Category 1 Credit*(s)™. Physicians should claim only the credit commensurate with the extent of their participation in the activity.

All other health care professionals requesting continuing education credit for this enduring material will be issued a certificate of participation.

DISCLOSURE OF CONFLICTS OF INTEREST
The EOCME assesses conflict of interest with its instructors, faculty, planners, and other individuals who are in a position to control the content of CME activities. All relevant conflicts of interest that are identified are thoroughly vetted by EOCME for fair balance, scientific objectivity, and patient care recommendations. EOCME is committed to providing its learners with CME activities that promote improvements or quality in healthcare and not a specific proprietary business or a commercial interest.

The planning committee, staff, authors and editors listed below have identified no financial relationships or relationships to products or devices they or their spouse/life partner have with commercial interest related to the content of this CME activity:
Amiethab Aiyer, MD; Peter J. Apel, MD, PhD; Chukwudi Chukwunyerenwa, MD; P. Christopher Cook, MD, FRCS; Andrew G. Georgiadis, MD; Jennifer Harrington, MBBS, FRACP; Kristen Helm; Willian Hennrikus, MD; Kerry Holland; Andrew W. Howard, MD, FRCSC, MSc; Brynne Hunter; Indu Kumari; Sandy Lavery; Jill McNair; James F. Mooney, III, MD; Lindsay Parnell; Richard Schwend, MD; Lee S. Segal, MD; Brian A. Shaw, MD; Etienne Sochett, MB ChB, FRCPC; Bonita F. Stanton, MD; Megan Suermann; Ira Zaltz, MD.

The planning committee, staff, authors and editors listed below have identified financial relationships or relationships to products or devices they or their spouse/life partner have with commercial interest related to the content of this CME activity:
Ron El-Hawary, MD is a consultant/advisor for and has a research gramt from Depuy Synthes Companies and Medtronic of Canada Ltd; also is a consultant/advisor for Halifax Biomedical Inc.
Brian Giordano, MD has research grants from Arthrex, Inc. and Carticept Medical, Inc.; also is a consultant/advisor for Arthrex, Inc.
Yi-Meng Yen, MD, PhD, MS is a consultant/advisor for OrthoPediatrics Corp., Smith & Nephew plc and Arthrex, Inc.

UNAPPROVED/OFF-LABEL USE DISCLOSURE
The EOCME requires CME faculty to disclose to the participants:
1. When products or procedures being discussed are off-label, unlabelled, experimental, and/or investigational (not US Food and Drug Administration [FDA] approved); and
2. Any limitations on the information presented, such as data that are preliminary or that represent ongoing research, interim analyses, and/or unsupported opinions. Faculty may discuss information about pharmaceutical agents that is outside of FDA-approved labelling. This information is intended solely for CME and is not intended to promote off-label use of these medications. If you have any questions, contact the medical affairs department of the manufacturer for the most recent prescribing information.

TO ENROLL

To enroll in the *Pediatric Clinics of North America* Continuing Medical Education program, call customer service at 1-800-654-2452 or sign up online at http://www.theclinics.com/home/cme. The CME program is available to subscribers for an additional annual fee of USD $290.

METHOD OF PARTICIPATION

In order to claim credit, participants must complete the following:

1. Complete enrolment as indicated above.
2. Read the activity.
3. Complete the CME Test and Evaluation. Participants must achieve a score of 70% on the test. All CME Tests and Evaluations must be completed online.

CME INQUIRIES/SPECIAL NEEDS

For all CME inquiries or special needs, please contact elsevierCME@elsevier.com.

Contributors

CONSULTING EDITOR

BONITA F. STANTON, MD
Vice Dean for Research and Professor of Pediatrics, School of Medicine, Wayne State University, Detroit, Michigan

EDITOR

P. CHRISTOPHER COOK, MD, FRCS(C)
Associate Professor, Division of Pediatric Orthopaedics, Department of Orthopaedics, Golisano Childrens Hospital, University of Rochester, Rochester, New York

AUTHORS

AMIETHAB AIYER, MD
Chief Resident, Department of Orthopaedic Surgery, Penn State College of Medicine, Hershey, Pennsylvania

PETER J. APEL, MD, PhD
Orthopaedics, Guthrie, Corning, New York

CHUKWUDI CHUKWUNYERENWA, MD, MCh, FRCS(C)
Paediatric Orthopaedic Fellow, IWK Health Center, Halifax, Nova Scotia, Canada

P. CHRISTOPHER COOK, MD, FRCS(C)
Associate Professor, Division of Pediatric Orthopaedics, Department of Orthopaedics, Golisano Childrens Hospital, University of Rochester, Rochester, New York

RON EL-HAWARY, MD, MSc, FRCS(C)
Chief of Orthopaedic Surgery, IWK Health Center; Associate Professor, Department of Surgery, Dalhousie University, Halifax, Nova Scotia, Canada

ANDREW G. GEORGIADIS, MD
Chief Resident, Department of Orthopaedic Surgery, Henry Ford Hospital, Detroit, Michigan

BRIAN D. GIORDANO, MD
Co-Director, Hip Preservation Program, Division of Sports Medicine; Assistant Professor, Department of Orthopaedics, University of Rochester, Rochester, New York

JENNIFER HARRINGTON, MBBS, FRACP
Division of Endocrinology, Department of Pediatrics, Hospital for Sick Children, University of Toronto, Toronto, Ontario, Canada

WILLIAM HENNRIKUS, MD
Professor of Orthopaedics and Associate Dean of Education, Department of Orthopaedic Surgery, Penn State College of Medicine, Hershey, Pennsylvania

ANDREW HOWARD, MD, MSc, FRCSC
Associate Professor, Division of Orthopedic Surgery, Department of Surgery, Hospital for Sick Children, University of Toronto, Toronto, Ontario, Canada

JAMES F. MOONEY III, MD
Chief, Pediatric Orthopaedic Surgery, Department of Orthopaedic Surgery, Medical University of South Carolina, Charleston, South Carolina

RICHARD M. SCHWEND, MD, FAAP
Professor, Orthopaedics and Pediatrics, The University of Missouri-Kansas City, Kansas City Medical Center, Kansas City, Missouri

LEE S. SEGAL, MD
Professor, Department of Orthopaedics, University of Wisconsin Hospital and Clinics, University of Wisconsin, Madison, Wisconsin

BRIAN A. SHAW, MD, FAAP, FAAOS
Associate Professor, Orthopaedic Surgery, University of Colorado School of Medicine, Children's Hospital Colorado and Memorial Health System, Colorado Springs, Colorado

ETIENNE SOCHETT, MB ChB, FRCPC
Division of Endocrinology, Department of Pediatrics, Hospital for Sick Children, University of Toronto, Toronto, Ontario, Canada

YI-MENG YEN, MD, PhD
Assistant Professor in Orthopaedic Surgery, Division of Sports Medicine, Boston Children's Hospital, Harvard Medical School, Boston, Massachusetts

IRA ZALTZ, MD
Associate Professor, Orthopaedic Surgery, William Beaumont Hospital, Royal Oak, Michigan

Contents

 Video of the Ortolani maneuver accompanies this article

> Developmental dysplasia of the hip (DDH) encompasses a spectrum of
> physical and imaging findings. The child's hip will not develop normally if
> it remains unstable and anatomically abnormal by walking age. Therefore,
> careful physical examination of all infants to diagnose and treat significant
> DDH is critical to provide the best possible functional outcome. Regard-
> less of the practice setting, all health professionals who care for newborns
> and infants should be trained to evaluate the infant hip for instability and to
> provide appropriate and early conservative treatment or referral.

> Transient synovitis, septic hip, and Legg-Calvé-Perthes disease are com-
> mon conditions in children. Distinguishing between these disorders can be
> a diagnostic challenge. Similar presentations, in an age group difficult to
> examine, coupled with literature that is confusing creates difficulty. It is
> important to make the correct diagnosis of septic hip in a timely fashion
> to avoid serious and potentially crippling consequences. As there is no
> single test for discriminating between these conditions, knowledge of
> the nuances of clinical presentation, physical examination, laboratory
> investigations, and imaging is essential. Judicious use of clinical algo-
> rithms can complement clinical acumen.

> Slipped capital femoral epiphysis (SCFE) involves displacement of the
> proximal femoral metaphysis relative to a fixed epiphysis, usually during
> a period of rapid growth and unique physeal susceptibility. Patients have
> characteristic clinical, histologic, and radiologic features. Several clinical
> signs and medical diagnoses should prompt radiologic and laboratory
> workup. Limp or hip or knee pain in a patient 10 to 16 years old should
> include SCFE in the differential. If confirmed, appropriate treatment

involves proximal femoral physeal stabilization and/or realignment. The optimal surgical treatment of severe SCFE and its late sequela remain an evolving and controversial subject.

Brian D. Giordano

 A video of Impingement and instability testing accompanies this article

Hip pain in the adolescent athlete is a common source of functional impairment and can limit athletic performance. In the past, many intra- and extra-articular hip abnormalities went unrecognized and were left untreated because of insufficient diagnostic imaging and limited surgical options. However, over the past 20 years, there has been a tremendous expansion research, and the understanding of the etiology of hip pain among such athletes has grown. Improvements in imaging modalities and technical innovations have led to greater diagnostic insights and creative new treatment strategies. This article explores the etiology and treatment of hip pain in the adolescent athlete.

Yi-Meng Yen

Knee pain in children and adolescents is one of the most prevalent complaints in a pediatric practice, accounting for at least a third of musculoskeletal complaints. Accurate diagnosis requires an understanding of knee anatomy and patterns of knee injuries and skill in physical examination. This review covers the most common causes of knee pain in children and adolescents, including overuse issues, such as Osgood-Schlatter and osteochondritis dissecans, as well as traumatic injuries, including tibial spine fractures and anterior cruciate ligament injuries.

James F. Mooney III

Familial concern regarding perceived rotational and angular deformities is a common part of any primary care practice. It is essential for the medical practitioner to understand the wide normal range in children and the natural history of lower extremity development over time. Most lower extremity rotational and angular issues in young children resolve spontaneously over time, and require little or no intervention. In the current atmosphere of medical cost containment, coupled with the shortage of pediatric orthopedic surgeons, many of these patients should be managed by the primary care provider and do not require referral for more specialized care.

Amiethab Aiyer and William Hennrikus

There are multiple causes of pediatric foot and ankle pain. Although conservative measures are appropriate for initial management, patients with refractory pain should be given consideration for further intervention. This review highlights some of the most common causes of foot and ankle pain in the child, with specific attention to demographics, etiologies, diagnostic workup, and treatment options.

Pediatric Orthopedics

PEDIATRIC CLINICS OF NORTH AMERICA

DOWNLOAD
Free App!

Review Articles
THE CLINICS

NOW AVAILABLE FOR YOUR iPhone and iPad

Foreword

Pediatric Orthopedics

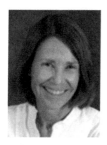

Bonita F. Stanton, MD
Consulting Editor

Among the many important decisions that general pediatricians must make on a daily basis are those depending on the recognition of conditions requiring timely referral to pediatric orthopedic surgeons. This year the Surgical Advisory Panel of the American Academy of Pediatrics issued an important policy statement identifying a range of conditions requiring timely referral to pediatric surgical specialists, including pediatric orthopedic surgeons.[1] At the same time, it is equally important that pediatricians receive the training to recognize those disorders that they can—and should—be comfortable handling without involving pediatric orthopedic specialists. Such competence at the primary care level is important for the child, for his or her family, for the pediatrician, and for the pediatric orthopedic specialist.[2]

Over the past decade, several surveys of children referred by pediatricians to pediatric orthopedic surgeons have found evidence suggesting that approximately half of such referrals are inconsistent with the guidelines recommended by the Surgery Advisory Panel of the American Academy of Pediatrics[2,3]; that is, about half of the children referred had conditions that pediatricians should be comfortable assessing and managing.

It is the purpose of this issue to review conditions that are likely to present to pediatricians to update them as to the appropriate evaluation and treatment algorithm—including both management in their own offices and appropriate referrals. The articles in this issue are written for pediatricians and therefore are centered on the symptoms and concerns that might bring the child to their attention. The articles provide guidance as to the workup and evaluation of these children, including guidance as to what conditions and findings or constellations thereof need to be referred

Pediatr Clin N Am 61 (2014) xi–xii
http://dx.doi.org/10.1016/j.pcl.2014.09.002
0031-3955/14/$ – see front matter © 2014 Published by Elsevier Inc.

and when. It provides insightful guidance combining practical advice and major advances in the field.

Bonita F. Stanton, MD
School of Medicine
Wayne State University
1261 Scott Hall
540 East Canfield, Suite 1261
Detroit, MI 48201, USA

E-mail address:
bstanton@med.wayne.edu

REFERENCES

1. AAP Surgical Advisory Panel. Policy Statement: Referral to Pediatric Surgical Specialists. Pediatrics 2014;133(2):350–6.
2. Hsu EY, Schwend RM, Julia L. How many referrals to a pediatric orthopaedic hospital specialty clinic are primary care problems? J Pediatr Orthop 2012; 32(7):732–6.
3. Reeder BM, Lyne ED, Patel DR, et al. Referral patterns to a pediatric orthopedic clinic: implications for education and practice. Pediatrics 2004;113(3 Pt 1):e163–7.

Preface

Pediatric Orthopedics for the Primary Care Provider

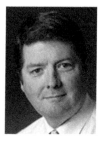

P. Christopher Cook, MD, FRCS(C)
Editor

It has been a great pleasure to help compile this Pediatric Orthopedic issue of the *Pediatric Clinics of North America*. Pediatric orthopedics has traditionally been a large part of the practice of a primary pediatric provider. Approximately 30% of problems encountered in a primary pediatric practice are related to the musculoskeletal system.[1] It is second only to ophthalmology as the most common subspecialty referral.[2] The American Academy of Pediatrics guidelines recommend that cases across a very broad range of diagnoses be referred to a pediatric orthopedic surgeon.[3] These diagnoses include benign bone tumors, congenital malformations, limb deformities, metabolic bone disease, infections of the bone and joints, hip dysplasia, and others. Large numbers of musculoskeletal patients carrying a very broad range of diagnoses, coupled with a traditional perception that orthopedic education in pediatric residency is limited, makes the evaluation, treatment, and referral of these conditions often confusing and difficult. This is thought to be part of the reason that 50% of referrals to pediatric orthopedists are primary care pediatric orthopedics cases.[4]

It is not the intention of this issue to provide an exhaustive document on the details of treatment (operative and nonoperative) of complex pediatric orthopedic problems. Rather, it is meant to afford the pediatric primary provider with updated information and a review of common pediatric orthopedic issues seen in the primary care office. In addition, it is intended to provide information of when to refer many of these conditions and to clarify some of the common confusions and controversies that exist.

In accordance with these principles, a survey of some pediatricians, pediatric orthopedic surgeons, and pediatric residents was completed to determine what might be the appropriate focus of the issue and the best topics to include. As a result, issues related to trauma that might be treated in the office, new diagnoses and treatments for hip pain in the adolescent, difficulties of knee pain, a myriad of foot problems, the natural history of rotational and angular deformities, and the difficulty in differentiating causes of hip irritability in young children were thought to be important to include.

Pediatr Clin N Am 61 (2014) xiii–xiv
http://dx.doi.org/10.1016/j.pcl.2014.09.001
0031-3955/14/$ – see front matter © 2014 Elsevier Inc. All rights reserved.

The intention is to help the primary care provider not only evaluate and treat these office conditions but also develop a sense of when to refer these patients.

Pediatric orthopedics is a very large diverse subspecialty. It has patients that range in age from 0 to 16 to 18 years. It deals with a very broad array of conditions that often affect more than the musculoskeletal system, and has patients that range from the elite athlete to those that are severely disabled and bedridden. It is hoped that this issue will help clinicians with their early evaluation and management of many of these common pediatric orthopedic conditions.

P. Christopher Cook, MD, FRCS(C)
Golisano Children's Hospital
University of Rochester
601 Elmwood Avenue
Box 665
Rochester, NY 14642, USA

E-mail address:
Christopher_Cook@URMC.Rochester.edu

REFERENCES

1. Schwend RM, Geiger J. Outpatient pediatric orthopedics: common and important conditions. Pediatr Clin North Am 1998;45:943–71.
2. Vernacchio L, Muto JM, Young G, et al. Ambulatory subspecialty visits in a large pediatric primary care network. Health Serv Res 2012;47(4):1755–69.
3. Surgical Advisory Panel. Guidelines for referral to pediatric surgical specialists. Pediatrics 2002;110:187–91.
4. Hsu EY, Schwend RM, Leamon J. How many referrals to a pediatric orthopaedic hospital specialty clinic are primary care problems? J Pediatr Orthop 2012; 32(7):727–31.

Evaluation and Treatment of Developmental Hip Dysplasia in the Newborn and Infant

Richard M. Schwend, MD[a], Brian A. Shaw, MD[b],*, Lee S. Segal, MD[c]

KEYWORDS

- Developmental hip dysplasia • Acetabular dysplasia • Hip subluxation
- Hip dislocation • Ortolani maneuver • Swaddling

KEY POINTS

- Research over the past decade has reinforced most of the principles and recommendations of the 2000 American Academy of Pediatrics' *Clinical Practice Guideline: Early Detection of Developmental Dysplasia of the Hip*.
- A reasonable goal for the primary care physician should be to prevent hip subluxation or dislocation by 6 months of age using the periodic examination.
- The Ortolani maneuver, in which a subluxated or dislocated femoral head is *gently* reduced into the acetabulum with hip abduction by the examiner, is the most important clinical test for detecting dysplasia in the newborn.
- Safe swaddling, in which the hips are not extended and does not restrict hip motion, does not increase the risk for developmental hip dysplasia.
- Despite best practice, young adults will still present with hip dysplasia that was not detected at birth.

 Video of the Ortolani maneuver accompanies this article at http://www.pediatric.theclinics.com/

INTRODUCTION

Developmental dysplasia of the hip (DDH) encompasses a spectrum of physical and imaging findings, ranging from mild temporary instability to frank dislocation. The

Disclosure: none.
[a] Orthopaedics and Pediatrics, UMKC, KUMC Director of Research Children's Mercy Hospital, 2401 Gillham Road, Kansas City, MO 64108, USA; [b] Orthopaedic Surgery, University of Colorado School of Medicine, Children's Hospital Colorado and Memorial Health System, Colorado Springs, 4125 Briargate Parkway, Suite 100, Colorado Springs, CO 80920, USA; [c] Department of Orthopaedics, University of Wisconsin Hospital and Clinics, University of Wisconsin, 1685 Highland Avenue, Room 6170-110, Madison, WI 53705-2281, USA
* Corresponding author.
E-mail address: coloradobonedoc@aol.com

Pediatr Clin N Am 61 (2014) 1095–1107
http://dx.doi.org/10.1016/j.pcl.2014.08.008
0031-3955/14/$ – see front matter © 2014 Elsevier Inc. All rights reserved.

child's hip will not develop normally if it remains unstable and anatomically abnormal by walking age. Therefore, careful physical examination of all infants to diagnosis and treat significant DDH is critical to provide the best possible functional outcome. Regardless of the practice setting, all health professionals who care for newborns and infants should be trained to evaluate the infant hip for instability and provide appropriate and early conservative treatment or referral. Unfortunately, musculoskeletal training in primary care residency programs and postgraduate education has received less attention than the prevalence of the condition warrants. Despite a normal newborn and infant hip examination, a late-onset hip dislocation still occurs in approximately 1 in 5000 infants as well as dysplasia in young adults.

INCIDENCE AND RISK FACTORS

The incidence of DDH varies from 1.5 to 25.0 per 1000 live births, depending on the criteria used for diagnosis, the population studied, and the method of screening. Relative risk rates are stated in the American Academy of Pediatrics' (AAP) 2000 clinical practice guidelines, and the overall DDH risk is about 1 per 1000. Traditional risk factors for DDH include breech position, female sex, being the first born, and a positive family history. Breech presentation is probably the most important single risk factor, with DDH reported in 2% to 20% of male and female infants presenting in the breech position.[1,2] Frank breech in a girl, with the hips flexed and knees extended, seems to have the highest risk. However, approximately 75% of DDH occurs in female infants without any other identified risk factors, so a careful physical examination of all infants' hips is required.[1]

The risk for DDH also depends on environmental factors. Newborn infants have hip and knee flexion contractures because of their normal intrauterine position. These contractures resolve over time with normal developmental maturation. Animal studies have shown that forced hip and knee extension in the neonatal period leads to hip dysplasia and dislocation because of increased tension in the hamstring and iliopsoas muscles that stresses the hip capsule, which may have underlying laxity or instability.[3] Comprehensive ultrasound screening during the immediate newborn period has demonstrated hip laxity in approximately 15% of infants.[4,5] The combination of capsular laxity and abnormal muscle tension is the most likely mechanism of DDH for infants who are maintained with the lower extremities extended and wrapped tightly together. In contrast, cultures that carry their children in the straddle or jockey position, common in warmer climates, have very low rates of hip dislocation compared with cultures that wrap their infants tightly with the lower limbs together and extended (**Fig. 1**).[6]

NATURAL HISTORY

The natural history of mild dysplasia and instability noted in the first few weeks of life is typically benign, with up to 88% resolving by 8 weeks of age.[7] However, the natural history of a child's hip that remains subluxated or dislocated by walking age is poor. Normal development of the hip joint depends on a femoral head that is stable and concentrically reduced in the acetabulum, a requirement for both to form spherically. Looseness or laxity within the acetabulum is termed *instability*. A nonconcentric position is termed *subluxation*. The deformity of the femoral head and acetabulum is termed *dysplasia*. With dislocation or severe subluxation, during the second half of infancy and beyond, limited hip abduction occurs, which the parent may notice during diaper change. As the child reaches walking age, a limp and lower-limb-length discrepancy may be apparent.

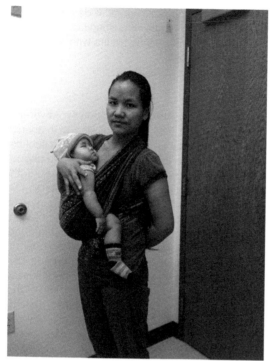

Fig. 1. A 10-month-old infant positioned in front of mother with her hips widely abducted. This position is safe for the hips, avoids stresses that could cause the hip to dislocate or subluxate, and encourages stable and concentric hip development.

With maturity and later in adulthood, patients may develop pain and degenerative arthritis in the hip, knee, and low back. Hip dysplasia, subluxation, and dislocation each have their own natural history. Subluxation may not be as well tolerated as dislocation if arthritis develops in early adulthood from excessive cartilage contact pressure. A completely dislocated hip with the femoral head located in the soft tissue may not cause functional problems other than knee or back pain or limp with limb-length discrepancy if the dislocation is unilateral. Completely dislocated hips, if bilateral with the femoral heads located in the soft tissues, may lead to severe waddling gait but can likewise be surprisingly pain free. Dislocated hips in which the femoral head cartilage is in contact with the bony pelvis may develop early arthritis by the fourth or later decades because of excessive wear of the femoral head cartilage on the pelvic bone. When arthritis develops in early adulthood, the burden of disability is high, with many requiring complex hip replacement at an early age. Over time, other diseases of the hip may occur and confound the natural history and outcome. These diseases includes trauma to the hip, infection, sickle cell disease, Perthes disease, slipped capital femoral epiphysis, and tuberculosis in resource-poor countries.[8]

SCREENING FOR DEVELOPMENTAL DYSPLASIA OF THE HIP

Screening for DDH is important because the condition may be initially occult, is easily treated when caught early, but difficult to treat later. When detected late, it may lead to long-term disability. Although detection in the neonatal period is ideal, a reasonable goal is to detect the subluxated or dislocated hip by 6 months of age. The physical examination is by far the most important means of detection. Radiography or sonography imaging should be used to confirm the suspicion of DDH. Despite all current methods of screening for DDH, most young adults with dysplasia who require a hip arthroplasty are not detected at birth.[9]

PHYSICAL EXAMINATION

A proper examination of infants includes observation for lower-limb-length discrepancy, asymmetric thigh or gluteal folds, Ortolani sign or maneuver, and limited or asymmetric abduction.[10] The Ortolani maneuver, in which a subluxated or dislocated femoral head is *gently* reduced into the acetabulum with hip abduction by the examiner, is the most important clinical test for detecting dysplasia in the newborn.[11] The Ortolani maneuver is a continuous smooth examination starting with the hip flexed and adducted with gentle anterior pressure on the trochanter followed by gently abducting the hip while sensing (termed *Segno dello scotto*) whether the hip slips into the acetabulum over the hypertrophied articular cartilage (Video 1). It answers the essential question: Is the femoral head dislocated and can it be reduced into the acetabulum? The examiner should not forcefully attempt to dislocate the femoral head. Although the Ortolani sign represents the palpable sensation of the femoral head moving into the acetabulum over the hypertrophied rim of the acetabular cartilage (termed the *neolimbus*), isolated high-pitched clicks represent the movement of myofascial tissues from the trochanter, knee, or other soft tissue.[12]

By about 3 months of age, a dislocated hip may become less mobile on physical examination, thus, limiting the usefulness and sensitivity of the Ortolani maneuver. However, at this time, restricted, asymmetric hip abduction becomes an important finding of hip dysplasia. Diagnosing bilateral DDH in older infants can be difficult because of the symmetry present when there is bilateral limited hip abduction. Other signs of a dislocated hip that are noticeable as infants reach walking age are a proximal thigh crease, a positive Galeazzi sign (in which the hips and knees are flexed 90° and the knee on the dislocated side appears lower), a wider-appearing perineum, a more prominent hip curvature, and a more proximally located posterior knee crease. By walking age, infants may have a delay in walking, a Trendelenburg limp, and a bilateral waddling gait if both hips are dislocated. On the other hand, mild hip dysplasia may have no symptoms or physical findings in infants or older children.

RADIOGRAPHY

Plain radiography becomes most useful by 4 to 6 months of age, when the femoral head's secondary center of ossification (ossific nucleus) forms, a finding that occurs earlier in female infants.[13] A single anteroposterior (AP) view of the entire pelvis is obtained, with positioning of the pelvis without rotation (**Fig. 2**). Acetabular dysplasia, subluxation, and dislocation are easily detected on the radiographs if taken after the femoral head's ossific nucleus has appeared. If subluxation or dislocation is noted, an AP view of the pelvis with the hips abducted can be done to document hip reducibility. However, there is debate whether minor radiographic variability in young infants (increased acetabular index) constitutes actual disease.[14] Radiographic hip screening is traditionally indicated for infants with risk factors, such as a history of breech presentation or an abnormal physical examination at 4 months of age.[2,10,15,16] An AP radiograph of the pelvis is obtained in newborns or infants if other conditions, such as congenital short femur, proximal focal femoral deficiency, septic hip infection, or coxa vara, are suspected.

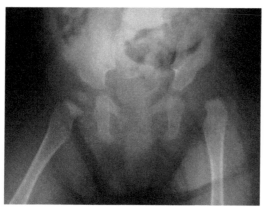

Fig. 2. AP radiograph of a 6-month-old infant. Note the dysplasia of the left hip with delayed ossific nucleus, superior and lateral dislocation, and small steep acetabulum.

ULTRASONOGRAPHY

The American Institute of Ultrasound in Medicine (AIUM) and the American College of Radiology (ACR) have published a joint guideline for the standardized performance of the infantile hip ultrasound.[17] Ultrasonography can provide detailed *static* and *dynamic* imaging of the hip before femoral head ossification. Ultrasound hip imaging can be *universal* for all infants or *selective* for those at risk for having DDH. Because disease prevalence is low at 1% to 2%, universal ultrasound screening is not generally practiced in North America or in countries with limited resources. Many barriers to successful ultrasound screening programs in the United States include expense, lack of availability, lack of trained personnel to assure quality imaging and interpretation, inconvenience, subjectivity, a high false-positive rate, and controversy about effectiveness.

Universal ultrasound screening of all infants is practiced in many European countries, with programs typically showing a decrease in the number of hips needing surgical reduction after their programs were begun. Most recently, a large randomized controlled study of universal or selective ultrasound screening in Norway that was compared with a well-done physical examination showed higher treatment rates but no significant decrease in late cases of DDH.[18] This same group of patients who underwent ultrasound screening and were followed to skeletal maturity did not have less acetabular dysplasia or degenerative change, although there was also no increased rate of avascular necrosis.[18] Despite this screening program for DDH, 92% of young adults with hip dysplasia who required a total hip arthroplasty were not detected at birth.[9] Results of these quality studies indicate that a well-performed physical examination in infants is the most important means of detecting instability; however, dysplasia is currently undetectable at birth for many adults.

In countries with very limited resources, even *selective* ultrasound screening is not typically available. The lack of ultrasound screening in low-income countries does not necessarily restrict the delivery of quality care for detecting and treating DDH. In these countries, primary prevention through education about proper swaddling, early detection with a properly performed physical examination by trained health care workers and early safe conservative treatment are the basis of an effective DDH program. Similar to the emphasis on conservative clubfoot treatment in countries with limited resources, education, primary prevention, early detection and treatment are need to be developed (http://hipdysplasia.org). Despite successful early prevention, undetected genetically determined acetabular dysplasia may still present in the young adult.[19]

Ultrasound *screening* should *not* be performed before 3 to 4 weeks of age in infants with clinical signs or risk factors for DDH because of the normal physiologic laxity that typically resolves by 6 weeks of age.[17] Most minor sonographic hip anomalies seen at 4 weeks to 4 months of age will resolve spontaneously. These anomalies include minor changes in morphology and subluxation (*uncoverage*) with stress maneuvers. Proper timing, performance, and interpretation of infantile hip ultrasound imaging per the guidelines of the AIUM and the ACR is critical to avoid undertreatment or overtreatment. If available, ultrasound imaging can be used to guide the reduction of a dislocated hip in infants who are being treated in a Pavlik harness or other hip abduction orthosis (**Fig. 3**). With the current medicolegal climate that fosters defensive medicine, widespread ultrasonography has become the default ordered test, resulting in excessive referral and treatment as well as poor use of limited resources for infants with very mild dysplasia or laxity.[20,21] Developing local/regional criteria for screening imaging and referral based on best resources, especially for ultrasonography, should promote more uniform and cost-effective treatment.

SWADDLING

Traditional swaddling that is still practiced in many cultures with the lower extremities fully extended and wrapped together can cause hip subluxation and dislocation (**Fig. 4**). Studies of Native Americans before the 1950s demonstrated a very high prevalence of hip dislocation in communities when their babies were carried on a cradleboard with the hips and knees strapped in an extended and adducted position. The frequency of childhood hip dislocation decreased dramatically among Navajo infants after cloth diapers were introduced. This decrease in the incidence of hip dislocation

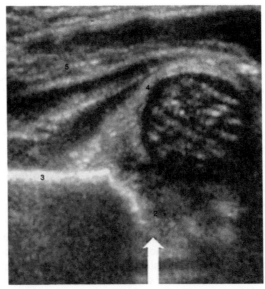

Fig. 3. Ultrasound of hip. (1) Femoral head, (2) acetabulum, (3) lateral border of ilium, (4) labrum, (5) abductor muscles. Arrow points to the triradiate cartilage.

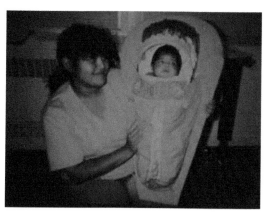

Fig. 4. Infant in traditional cradleboard. Infants would spend much of their time in this devise with hips tightly bound. Over time, the swaddling has become less tight; infants now wear diapers, and time in the cradleboard has decreased in favor of car seats and other carriers. As a result, the prevalence of DDH in the Navajo population, which previously was 6 times the US national average, is now similar.

among Navajo infants was attributed to the slightly flexed and abducted position from the bulky cloth diapers even when the infants were strapped on the cradleboard. Recently, as the frequency of cradleboard use and time spent in the cradleboard in Navajo society has diminished, so has the prevalence of hip dysplasia, from a rate of 6 times the US average to a prevalence similar to the rest of the US population. A similar experience has been documented in Japan where the incidence of DDH was 1.5% to 3.5% before 1965. Following the implementation of a national program to eliminate swaddling with the hips and knees in an extended position, the incidence of DDH decreased to 0.2%.[3] A significant relationship between swaddling and hip dysplasia was also identified in Turkey.[22] Although the frequency of traditional swaddling has been reduced in Turkey, traditional swaddling during infancy is still the greatest risk factor compared with breech birth, family history, or sex.[23] A systematic review of swaddling noted that DDH is more prevalent when the lower limbs are bound so they are not free to move.[24]

Despite the known risks to the tightly bound hip, swaddling has grown in popularity among parents in the United States and internationally. The concept of safe swaddling, which does not restrict hip motion but rather allows the hips to remain in the human or naturally flexed and abducted position, has been shown to lessen the risk of DDH.[24–31] The International Hip Dysplasia Institute and the Pediatric Orthopedic Society of North America have issued the following statement about the safety of swaddling:

Infant hips should be positioned in slight flexion and abduction during swaddling. The knees should also be maintained in slight flexion. Additional free movement in the direction of hip flexion and abduction may have some benefit [http:// hipdysplasia.org]. Avoidance of forced or sustained passive hip extension and adduction in the first few months of life is essential for proper hip development.

Contemporary methods of swaddling emphasize upper extremity wrapping while allowing ample room for hip and knee flexion (**Fig. 5**) (video available at http:// hipdysplasia.org/developmental-dysplasia-of-the-hip/hip-healthy-swaddling/).[32] Prevention of DDH should begin with encouragement of flexed and abducted hip

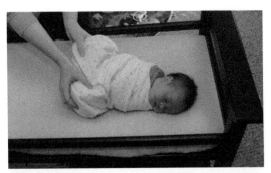

Fig. 5. Safe swaddling technique. Notice that while the upper extremities are securely wrapped, the hips and lower extremities are free to move with hip flexion and abduction.

positioning during early infancy in all infants. Infants who have been swaddled tightly with the hips and legs bound together in extension should have a focused attention to their periodic clinical hip examination and treating physicians need to have a frank discussion with their parents regarding safe swaddling technique.

TREATMENT

Early detection and referral of DDH allows appropriate intervention with bracing or casting, which, for most treated infants, may safely prevent the need for reconstructive surgery. It is likely that a primary care physician or health care worker will be the first to detect hip dysplasia, so all who care for newborns and infants in the primary care setting need proper training in the diagnosis and appropriate referral of these children. The physical examination, despite advances in ultrasound imaging, remains the most important screening tool, especially because most infants with DDH have no identified risk factors other than female sex.[33–35] In a study of children on the US Navajo Reservation that used the AAP's guidelines, most significant DDH was detected by a competent newborn physical examination performed by a pediatrician or general practitioner.[10,16] The more severe the instability, the more useful was the physical examination in detecting DDH.[36] In a decision analysis model, the lowest probability of developing degenerative disease of the hip by 60 years of age was doing a thorough physical examination of the hip on all newborns.[37]

Any infant with a positive Ortolani maneuver should be closely followed or referred for evaluation. An infant with a persistent positive Ortolani maneuver on repeat examination should be referred for treatment. An infant with limited or asymmetric abduction should receive an ultrasound examination if younger than 4 to 6 months, or a radiograph if older, with treatment provided for children with a dislocated or subluxated hip. Periodic physical examination should be performed and documented on all children until walking age.[10]

If the newborn hip is not clinically stable by 3 weeks of age, treatment with a hip abduction devise, such as a Pavlik harness or von Rosen splint, is recommended. These devices can be used for infants who are up to 6 months of age and are typically managed by an orthopedic surgeon who has training, interest, and expertise in DDH. The goal of treatment is to use an orthosis until the hip is documented by physical examination and ultrasound imaging to be stable. Serial ultrasonography and radiography are used by the treating orthopedist to determine the efficacy of treatment. If Pavlik harness treatment is used, precautions, such as avoiding forced abduction, stopping treatment after 3 weeks if the hip does not reduce, and proper strap placement with weekly monitoring, is important to minimize the small risks that are associated with this treatment. After the hip has become stable in the Pavlik harness, longer treatment with the harness or a hip abduction orthosis is typically used until the acetabulum morphology is normalized. The older the child is at the time of treatment, the longer treatment may assure stability and normalization of acetabular morphology. Although up to 90% of hips in newborns or young infants can be successfully treated with a Pavlik harness, not all hips become stable. Closed reduction and casting may be needed if the hip does not become stable by 3 weeks of Pavlik harness treatment.

After 6 months of age, surgical treatment with arthrogram, adductor tenotomy, and spica cast is an effective conservative approach for children with a dislocated hip to achieve a concentric closed reduction. After children have achieved walking ability, open reduction of the hip is often required because of the development of fixed contractures and deformity that respond less predictably to closed reduction. This procedure is specialized surgery and should be performed by an orthopedic surgeon with the appropriate level of training, experience, and expertise. The risks of bracing, casting, and surgical treatment may include avascular necrosis (AVN), nonconcentric reduction, redislocation, femoral nerve palsy, and obturator (inferior) hip dislocation.[38–40] The risk of AVN is higher in older children who need surgical treatment than with a conservative Pavlik harness or brace treatment in infants. The increased risk with late treatment compared with early treatment reinforces the principle of early screening and treatment over later surgical management. Regardless of the method used, reduction of the hip should never be forced or held in an extreme position.[41,42] Surgical treatment in the infant and young child has the added risks of anesthesia, infection, redislocation, stiffness and later arthritis. Long term, all children with a history of DDH should be followed until skeletal maturity.

In countries with limited resources, even in the United States or other developed countries, children may present with DDH after walking age. A 3-year-old child who presents with a unilateral dislocated hip may have a reasonable outcome after open reduction, femoral shortening, and acetabular osteotomy, if the surgery is precisely performed, the reduction is gentle and concentric, stability is maintained, and AVN is either avoided or minimalized. Although there is no exact age cutoff for when

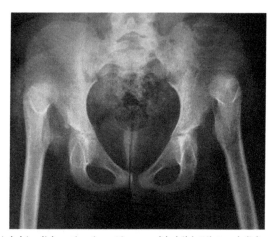

Fig. 6. Bilateral high hip dislocation in a 10-year-old child. Bilateral dislocations, because of symmetry, may be more difficult to detect in infants or young children. It is a reasonable goal for the primary care physician to prevent hip subluxation or dislocation by 6 months of age using the periodic examination.

children are too old for surgical treatment, as children become older than 3 years, results will deteriorate with increasing age of surgery.[43] Castaneda and colleagues[44] reported that the long-term results of Iowa Hip Score, PODCI (Pediatric Outcomes Data Collection Instrument), hip centering, and radiographic hip morphology diminished with the age at the time of surgery. A unilateral hip dislocation in a 5 year old with well-preserved hip morphology may do well if surgery is expertly performed. However, bilateral open hip reductions in an 8 year old with highly dysplastic acetabula and femoral heads will likely have poor long-term outcome from the surgery and is best left untreated (**Fig. 6**). Besides a generally worse outcome in older children, the additional complications of osteonecrosis and redislocation predict the poorest results.[43] Half of surgically reduced hips may still require further surgery. Even the opposite normal hip may eventually show significant dysplasia, suggesting a genetic cause. Once surgery

---

Box 1
Summary statement and recommendations

The following recommendations have been developed by the DDH Task Force of the AAP Section on Orthopedics:

1. Tight swaddling of the lower extremities with the hips extended should be avoided. The concept of safe swaddling, which does not restrict hip motion, minimizes the risk for DDH.

2. The AAP, the Pediatric Orthopaedic Society of North America, the American Academy of Orthopaedic Surgeons, and the Canadian DDH Task Force recommend newborn and periodic screening examinations for DDH to include evaluating for positive Ortolani maneuver in newborns and young infants, detection of limb-length discrepancy, asymmetric thigh or buttock (gluteal) creases, limited abduction (generally positive after 3 months of age) and associated findings of torticollis, ligamentous laxity, and foot deformity.

3. Evidence strongly supports screening for and *treatment* of hip *subluxation* and *dislocation* (Ortolani positive) and *observation* of milder early forms of dysplasia and instability (Barlow positive).

4. It is acceptable to refer children with suspected DDH or with positive risk factors to a pediatric orthopedist without a prior ultrasound, which is preferable to obtaining an improperly timed or poorly performed study.

5. Treatment of neonatal DDH is not an emergency. In-hospital initiation of bracing by the primary care physician or other health professional is not required if infants with persistent instability are referred to the orthopedic surgeon within several weeks. Initiation of treatment is based on the clinical examination of instability.

6. Ultrasonography can be useful between 4 weeks and 4 to 6 months of age for infants with risk factors for DDH. These risk factors include clinical instability, breech presentation, and positive family history. Other considerations for imaging studies, especially if there is a persistent concern about the clinical examination include first-born girls, parental concern, and a history of improperly performed lower extremity swaddling.

7. Radiography (AP and frog lateral pelvis views) is useful after 4 to 6 months of age for infants with risk factors or positive clinical findings. There is a period between 4 and 6 months of age when either a radiograph or ultrasound imaging can be used.

8. A reasonable goal for the primary care physician should be to prevent hip subluxation or dislocation by 6 months of age using the periodic examination. Selective ultrasonography or radiography is used in consultation with the pediatric radiologist and orthopedist. Screening programs have not completely eliminated the risk of a late presentation of DDH. Milder forms of dysplasia may resolve spontaneously or with early treatment. However, dysplasia that may require arthroplasty in young adults has not been completely prevented by screening and early treatment.

has failed and revision is contemplated, this repeat surgery in older children has very poor overall long-term results (**Box 1**).

SUPPLEMENTARY DATA

Supplementary data related to this article can be found online at http://dx.doi.org/10.1016/j.pcl.2014.08.008.

REFERENCES

1. Bache CE, Clegg J, Herron M. Risk factors for developmental dysplasia of the hip: ultrasonographic findings in the neonatal period. J Pediatr Orthop B 2002; 11(3):212–8.
2. Imrie M, Scott V, Stearns P, et al. Is ultrasound screening for DDH in babies born breech sufficient? J Child Orthop 2010;4(1):3–8.
3. Yamamuro T, Ishida K. Recent advances in the prevention, early diagnosis, and treatment of congenital dislocation of the hip in Japan. Clin Orthop Relat Res 1984;184:34–40.
4. Rosendahl K, Markestad T, Lie RT. Ultrasound screening for developmental dysplasia of the hip in the neonate: the effect on treatment rate and prevalence of late cases. Pediatrics 1994;94:47–52.
5. US Preventive Services Task Force. Screening for developmental dysplasia of the hip: recommendation statement. Pediatrics 2006;117:898–902.
6. Salter RB. Etiology, pathogenesis and possible prevention of congenital dislocation of the hip. Can Med Assoc J 1968;98:933–45.
7. Barlow TG. Early diagnosis and treatment of congenital dislocation of the hip. J Bone Joint Surg Br 1962;44B:292–301.
8. Oniankitan O, Kakpovi K, Flanyo E, et al. Risk factors for hip osteoarthritis in Lome, Togo. Med Trop (Mars) 2009;69(1):59–60.
9. Engesaeter IO, Lie SA, Lehmann TG, et al. Neonatal hip instability and risk of total hip replacement in young adulthood: follow-up of 2,218,596 newborns from the Medical Birth Registry of Norway in the Norwegian Arthroplasty Register. Acta Orthop 2008;79(3):321–6.
10. Committee on Quality Improvement, Subcommittee on Developmental Dysplasia of the Hip. American Academy of Pediatrics: clinical practice guideline: early detection of developmental dysplasia of the hip. Pediatrics 2000;105:896–905.
11. Lipton GE, Guille JT, Altiok H, et al. A reappraisal of the Ortolani examination in children with developmental dysplasia of the hip. J Pediatr Orthop 2007;27(1):27–31.
12. Bond CD, Hennrikus WL, DellaMaggiore ED. Prospective evaluation of newborn soft-tissue hip "clicks" with ultrasound. J Pediatr Orthop 1997;17(2):199–201.
13. Scoles PV, Boyd A, Jones PK. Radiographic parameters of the normal infant hip. J Pediatr Orthop 1987;7(6):656–63.
14. Mladenov K, Dora C, Wicart P, et al. Natural history of hips with borderline acetabular index and acetabular dysplasia in infants. J Pediatr Orthop 2002;22(5): 607–12.
15. Karmazyn BK, Gunderman RB, Coley BD, et al. American College of Radiology ACR Appropriateness Criteria on developmental dysplasia of the hip—child. J Am Coll Radiol 2009;6(8):551–7.
16. Schwend RM, Schoenecker P, Richards BS, et al. Pediatric Orthopaedic Society of North America Screening the newborn for developmental dysplasia of the hip: now what do we do? J Pediatr Orthop 2007;27:607–10.

17. American Institute of Ultrasound in Medicine, American College of Radiology. AIUM practice guideline for the performance of an ultrasound examination for detection and assessment of developmental dysplasia of the hip. J Ultrasound Med 2009;28(1):114–9.

18. Laborie LB, Engesaiter IO, Lehmann TG, et al. Screening strategies for hip dysplasia: long-term outcome of a randomized controlled trial. Pediatrics 2013; 132(3):492–501.

19. Schwend RM, Pratt WB, Fultz J. Untreated acetabular dysplasia of the hip in the Navajo. A 34 year case series follow-up. Clin Orthop Relat Res 1999;(364):108–16.

20. Elbourne D, Dezateux C, Arthur R, et al. Ultrasonography in the diagnosis and management of developmental hip dysplasia (UK Hip Trial): clinical and economic results of a multicentre randomized controlled trial. Lancet 2002;360(9350):2009–17.

21. Moore FH. Examining infants' hips – can it do harm? J Bone Joint Surg Br 1989; 71B:4–5.

22. Kutlu A, Memik R, Mutlu M, et al. Congenital dislocation of the hip and its relation to swaddling used in Turkey. J Pediatr Orthop 1992;12:598–602.

23. Dogruel H, Atalar H, Yavuz OY, et al. Clinical examination versus ultrasonography in detecting developmental dysplasia of the hip. Int Orthop 2008;32(3):415–9.

24. van Sleuwen BE, Engelberts AC, Boere-Boonekamp MM, et al. Swaddling: a systematic review. Pediatrics 2007;120:e1097–106.

25. Gerard CM, Harris KA, Thach BT. Physiologic studies on swaddling: an ancient child care practice, which may promote the supine position for infant sleep. J Pediatr 2002;141:398–403.

26. Mahan ST, Kasser JR. Does swaddling influence developmental dysplasia of the hip? Pediatrics 2008;121:177–8.

27. Oden RP, Powell C, Sims A, et al. Swaddling: will it get babies onto their backs for sleep? Clin Pediatr 2012;51:254–9.

28. Wang E, Liu T, Li J, et al. Does swaddling influence developmental dysplasia of the hip. J Bone Joint Surg Am 2012;94:1071–7.

29. International Hip Dysplasia Institute (Online resources). Available at: http://hipdysplasia.org. Accessed on July 1, 2014.

30. American Academy of Orthopaedic Surgeons (Online resources). Available at: http://orthoinfo.aaos.org/topic.cfm?topic=A00347. Accessed on July 1, 2014.

31. Pediatric Orthopaedic Society of North America (Online resources). Available at: http://posna.org/. Accessed on July 1, 2014.

32. Karp HN. Safe swaddling and healthy hips: don't toss the baby out with the bathwater. Pediatrics 2008;121:1075–6.

33. Jones DA. Neonatal hip stability and the Barlow test. J Bone Joint Surg Br 1991; 73B:216–8.

34. Patel H. Canadian Task Force on Preventive Health Care, 2001 update: screening and management of developmental dysplasia of the hip in newborns. Can Med Assoc J 2001;164:1669–77.

35. Shipman SA, Helfand M, Moyer VA, et al. Screening for developmental dysplasia of the hip: a systematic literature review for the U.S. Preventive Services Task Force. Pediatrics 2006;117:e557–76.

36. Schwend MR, Schooley A. The ship rock developmental dysplasia of the hip screening project. 37th Annual Carrie Tingley Winter Seminar. University of New Mexico. Albuquerque (New Mexico), February 2, 2007.

37. Mahan ST, Katz JN, Kim YJ. To screen or not to screen? A decision analysis of the utility of screening for developmental dysplasia of the hip. J Bone Joint Surg Am 2009;91(7):1705–19.

38. Suzuki S, Kashiwagi N, Kasahara Y, et al. Avascular necrosis and the Pavlik harness. The incidence of avascular necrosis in three types of congenital dislocation of the hip as classified by ultrasound. J Bone Joint Surg Br 1996;78(4):631–5.
39. Murnaghan ML, Browne RH, Sucato DJ, et al. Femoral nerve palsy in Pavlik harness treatment for developmental dysplasia of the hip. J Bone Joint Surg Am 2011;93(5):493–9.
40. Rombouts JJ, Kaelin A. Inferior (obturator) dislocation of the hip in neonates. A complication of treatment by the Pavlik harness. J Bone Joint Surg Br 1992; 74(5):708–10.
41. Kitoh H, Kawasumi M, Ishiguro N. Predictive factors for unsuccessful treatment of developmental dysplasia of the hip by the Pavlik harness. J Pediatr Orthop 2009; 29(6):552–7.
42. Mubarak S, Garfin S, Vance R, et al. Pitfalls in the use of the Pavlik harness for treatment of congenital dysplasia, subluxation, and dislocation of the hip. J Bone Joint Surg Am 1981;63(8):1239–48.
43. Holman J, Carrroll KL, Murray KA, et al. Long-term follow-up of open reduction surgery for developmental dislocation of the hip. J Pediatr Orthop 2012;32(2):121–4.
44. Castañeda P, Arana E, Haces F, et al. Functional and radiographic results of surgical treatment of patients with neglected developmental dysplasia of the hip. Albuquerque (New Mexico): POSNA; 2008.

Transient Synovitis, Septic Hip, and Legg-Calvé-Perthes Disease

An Approach to the Correct Diagnosis

P. Christopher Cook, MD, FRCS(C)

KEYWORDS

- Range of motion • Clinical algorithm • Effusion • Fever • Non–weight bearing

KEY POINTS

- The differentiation of septic hip from other inflammatory causes of hip pain in the child can be difficult.
- It is essential not to miss or delay the diagnosis of a septic hip.
- Using knowledge of the presentations of these diagnoses along with good clinical acumen, the physician can achieve these goals.
- It is very important to incorporate all information from the history, physical examination, laboratory tests, and imaging, with an emphasis on range of motion and the judicious use of clinical algorithms.

EPIDEMIOLOGY

Transient synovitis is a self-limited condition of unknown etiology.[1] There is some evidence linking it to a viral infection, but this has not been substantiated. There is often an antecedent upper respiratory infection that may be a predisposing factor, and it is one of the most common causes of painful (irritable) hip in childhood. Synovitis can occur in toddlers and in adolescence, but most patients are between 3 and 8 years with a mean age of 6 years. The right side is slightly more commonly involved, but bilateral synovitis has been reported. There is a male predilection (approximately 2:1).[2]

Septic arthritis is an orthopedic emergency. Purulent exudate is toxic to hyaline cartilage, and can damage or destroy a joint relatively quickly. Beginning treatment within 4 days from the initial onset of symptoms usually affords a good prognosis. Once frank purulence is established, however, the hip may be devastated in a matter

Disclosure: None.
Division of Pediatric Orthopaedics, Department of Orthopaedics, Golisano Childrens Hospital, University of Rochester, 601 Elmwod Avenue, Rochester, NY 14642, USA
E-mail address: Christopher_Cook@urmc.rochester.edu

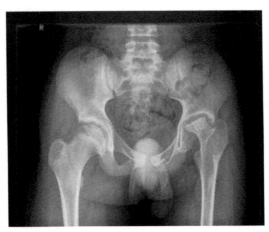

Fig. 1. Left hip shows loss of femoral epiphysis and severe destruction secondary to undiagnosed septic hip.

of hours. **Fig. 1** demonstrates the destruction that sepsis of the hip can cause when treated late. The joint can be infected through the hematogenous route, direct inoculation through trauma or surgery, and contiguous spread. In the case of the hip, the latter would be from osteomyelitis of the intra-articular portion of the femoral head and neck draining into the joint. This phenomenon is most common in the neonate and infant (**Fig. 2**). Septic arthritis has a similar age distribution but is perhaps more common when presenting at age less than 2 years. It is more common in boys than in girls, and can present in more than 1 joint at a time, although this is rare.[3]

Legg (United States), Calvé (France), and Perthes (Germany) described what is now known as Legg-Calvé-Perthes (LCP) disease independently in 1910.[4] The condition is initiated by the loss of blood flow to the femoral head. The subsequent healing brings on the clinical syndrome of pain, femoral head collapse, and eventual osteoarthritis. Despite much work and many theories, the etiology continues to be unknown, making treatment highly controversial. It is more common in boys and can be bilateral in 20%

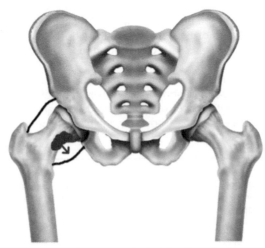

Fig. 2. Osteomyelitis of the right femoral neck draining into the hip causing septic arthritis.

to 30% of cases. Usually when bilateral the two sides present sequentially within 18 months, although bilateral LCP disease is uncommon. The age range is again similar to transient synovitis (3–10 years) but, unlike septic arthritis, it is more common in older children (6–8 years).

CLINICAL PRESENTATION

As noted, infants and young toddlers (<2 years) will tend to have septic arthritis. Children older than 9 years will be less likely to have septic arthritis or transient synovitis. The biggest diagnostic challenge is in the 3- to 8-year age range. It is not uncommon for any of these conditions to present during this time. Their presentations are very similar:

- Variable onset of hip pain
- Limp, refusal to bear weight
- Limitation of movement
- Fever

There are, however, some nuances that may be helpful in differentiation. Factors to consider include (**Table 1**):

- Trauma
  - Trauma is commonly noted in the history. It is a common occurrence at the beginning of symptoms in all 3 diagnoses, and should always be part of the differential. One must remember that more than 1 diagnosis may exist. Indeed, in young children the evaluation can be difficult. There are case reports of septic arthritis being mistaken for a toddler's fracture.[5] As a result of the way a toddler's fracture tends to spiral, the tenderness is most commonly at the junction of the middle and distal thirds of the tibia posteromedially. It may not be as tender anterolaterally.
- Onset
  - Differences in the onset can be helpful. A relatively short history of symptoms over a couple of days is common in septic arthritis and transient synovitis. One

Table 1
Differentiation of septic hip from other inflammatory causes of hip pain

	Transient Synovitis	Septic Hip	Legg-Calvé-Perthes Disease
Trauma	Mild at beginning of symptoms	Mild at beginning of symptoms	Less likely. May be some distance from onset of symptoms
Onset	Several days (3–5)	Several days (3–5)	Weeks/months/ intermittent
Fever	No. Sometimes low grade <38	Yes >38.5	No
Appears ill	No	Yes	No
Gait	Limp (sometimes not weight bearing)	Not weight bearing (sometimes limp)	Limp to normal gait
Pain	Mild to severe	Moderate to severe	Mild to moderate
Range of motion	Pain at the end of motion arc	Severe pain throughout motion arc	Guarding, with pain on flexion and internal rotation

must bear in mind that concomitant osteomyelitis or antibiotic treatment may mitigate the acute nature of the presentation of septic arthritis. A longer presentation (~10–14 days) with a more acute worsening over the previous couple of days may indicate an osteomyelitis that has seeded the joint. LCP disease tends to present over a longer period of time (weeks to months) and may even be intermittent in nature. Indeed, a recurrence of "transient synovitis" may indicate that the diagnosis is LCP disease. On occasion LCP can present with an acute irritable hip.

- Pain
  - Pain is a large part of all of these diagnoses, but severity may help in differentiation. Both sepsis and transient synovitis pain can be moderate to very severe. Pain alone does not differentiate between these 2 entities. Patients with LCP disease tend not to have severe pain and indeed may not have much pain at all. Nonsteroidal anti-inflammatory medications can help relieve the discomfort of transient synovitis, but tend to be ineffective in cases of septic hip.
  - Pain is usually felt in the groin region. Three nerves innervate the hip; therefore, the pain might radiate to the medial thigh (obturator nerve), the buttock (sciatic nerve), and the knee (femoral nerve). It is not uncommon for a child to undergo radiography and magnetic resonance imaging (MRI) of the knee when the problem is actually the hip. All skeletally immature individuals presenting with knee pain should, at least, have a thorough physical examination of the hip.
- Gait
  - Transient synovitis and septic arthritis both can present with refusal to bear weight, which would be distinctly unusual for LCP disease. All 3 might present with an antalgic gait (decreased stance phase on the affected side). LCP disease more commonly presents with a lurch (the body leans to the affected side during stance) or a stiff hip gait (the pelvis and lower back swing the whole leg through with little hip motion, instead of the hip flexors moving the hip to swing the leg through).
- Fever
  - A temperature greater than 38.5°C is not uncommon with septic arthritis, whereas a low-grade fever (<38°C) may be seen with transient synovitis. Fever is not a feature in the presentation of LCP disease.

CLASSIC/ARCHETYPAL EXAMINATION

It is accepted that the presentation and physical examination of these conditions lies across a spectrum. A more severe case of transient synovitis can be very similar to septic arthritis, whereas an early or partially treated case of septic hip can have the clinical appearance of transient synovitis.

In septic arthritis the child is febrile, appears ill, and is not animated, tending to lie still. There is no weight bearing. When there is a joint effusion, the joint will be held in a position that maximally increases the volume of the affected joint. The child will therefore posture the leg with the hip in slight flexion, abduction, and external rotation. Any motion, even a toggle of rotation of the hip, will be very painful.

A child with transient synovitis will look well, often playing with toys in the examination room but not moving the hip. There is no or, at most, low-grade fever (<38°C). There can be posturing of the hip but the pain on range of motion is less severe.

The child may refuse to walk but, unlike a patient with a septic hip, will commonly walk with a limp.

A child with LCP disease looks well and has no fever. The child is ambulatory and can have a limp, which may be subtle. There is little pain on motion of the hip but there is guarding of the hip while moving it. Pain is worse with flexion and internal rotation. This motion is the opposite of the direction the hip would take with an effusion. Pain on flexion and internal rotation is often the first evidence of irritability, and commonly is the last to resolve for all diagnoses.

Laboratory

Complete blood count (CBC), erythrocyte sedimentation rate (ESR), and C-reactive protein (CRP) constitute the typical blood work to be obtained (**Tables 2** and **3**).

Imaging

Several imaging modalities are available to investigate the child with an irritable hip.

Radiography

The best initial test is plain radiographs. An anteroposterior (AP) pelvis and bilateral frog-leg laterals (AP pelvis with the hips flexed and abducted into the frog position) should be ordered. A pelvic film is often more useful than a specific hip film because it not only allows for comparison with the other side but also provides information about the pelvis and sacroiliac joint that would otherwise not be identifiable (**Fig. 3**). All 3 diagnoses may have completely normal radiographs on initial presentation. Thus radiographs are taken not necessarily to differentiate between them but to rule out other causes of the pain, such as osteomyelitis, benign or malignant tumor, and trauma. Joint-space widening is often reported in this setting. Clinically, this is not a very helpful finding. It can be widened as a result of joint effusion in all 3 and is highly variable, being dependent on hip position and the angle of the radiograph.[6] The physician will already be suspicious of a hip effusion based on physical examination (posturing of hip and decreased motion with pain on internal rotation and flexion) (**Fig. 4**).

LCP disease will often have radiographic findings on initial presentation. Mild flattening of the femoral head, sclerosis, and a crescent sign may be present early on (**Fig. 5**).

Ultrasonography

Ultrasonography is a useful tool to identify whether there is an effusion. A bone to capsule distance of greater than 2 mm difference from side to side is considered an effusion (**Fig. 6**). There is some controversy as to whether ultrasonography can differentiate between septic and purulent effusions from an inflammatory effusion

Table 2 Complete blood count (CBC), erythrocyte sedimentation rate (ESR), and C-reactive protein (CRP) measures			
	Transient Synovitis	Septic Arthritis	Legg-Calvé-Perthes Disease
Fever	>38°C	>38.5°C	None
WBC ($\times 10^9$/L)	Normal <12	>12	Normal
ESR (mm/h)	<40	>40	Normal
CRP (mg/L)	Normal <20	>20	Normal

Table 3
Blood work levels for septic hip, transient synovitis, and LCP disease

	WBC ($\times 10^9$/L)	ESR (mm/h)	CRP (mg/L)
Septic arthritis	>12	>40	>20
Transient synovitis	Normal <12	Normal <40	Normal <20
LCP disease	Normal	Normal	Normal

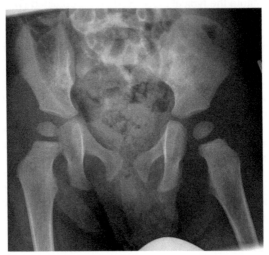

Fig. 3. AP pelvis showing a Salter Harris I fracture of the left proximal femoral physis. The physis is tilted compared to the left. This would be more difficult to pick up with only a x-ray of the left hip.

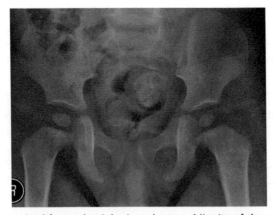

Fig. 4. A smaller proximal femoral epiphysis and some obliquity of the x-ray can make the joint space look large on the left. This patient did not have hip pain.

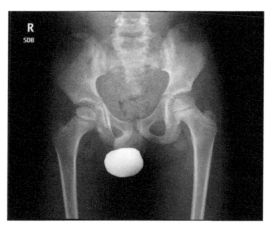

Fig. 5. Perthes disease of the right hip. Loss of epiphyseal height, lucency just under the joint line of the femoral head (crescent sign) and some flattening of the femoral head.

based on echogenicity. Therefore it should not be ordered to make or confirm the diagnosis of a septic hip.[7] It is very useful in assisting a hip aspiration. Using ultrasonography an aspiration can now be completed in the emergency department. A clinical evaluation of the fluid, stat Gram stain, and white blood cell count can be obtained and used to help determine whether formal drainage is necessary.[8,9]

Magnetic resonance imaging

The use of dynamic contrast-enhanced MRI has been reported and found to be able to differentiate between septic arthritis and transient synovitis,[10] although this modality is not widely used in the more acute setting. Time taken to reach the MRI scanner and the potential need for anesthetic in the younger child are detractors. In addition, unlike ultrasound-guided arthrocentesis, it does not provide a specimen. The best indication for MRI is in difficult cases after the acute issue of possible septic arthritis has been dealt with.

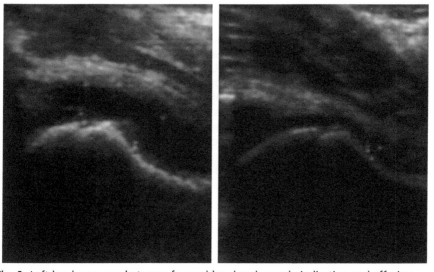

Fig. 6. Left has larger gap between femoral head and capsule indicating and effusion.

Bone scan

The use of a bone scan in this setting has largely been supplanted by ultrasonography and MRI. In the past, increased signal intensity on both sides of the joint and the amount of signal present in the femoral head were used to help make the diagnosis. The main use today is in the situation where clinical examination and other imaging methods have not been able to identify a pathologic area. A bone scan is fairly sensitive to blood flow, and can examine the whole body.

CLINICAL ALGORITHMS

In response to the difficulty in differentiating these diagnoses and the need to identify the potentially crippling disease of septic arthritis in an accurate and timely manner, much effort has been devoted to developing reliable clinical algorithms. In 1999 Kocher and colleagues[11] described an algorithm that determined the probability of septic arthritis using 4 clinical and laboratory markers/predictors.

Non–weight bearing	
Erythrocyte sedimentation rate (ESR)	$\geq$40 mm/h
White blood cell count (WBC)	$>12 \times 10^9$/L
Temperature	>38.5°C
Probability of Septic Arthritis	
Presence of 0 predictors	<0.2%
Presence of 1 predictor	3.0%
Presence of 2 predictors	40%
Presence of 3 predictors	93.1%
All 4 predictors present	99.6%

This tool has been beneficial in helping the physician make the correct clinical decision. Others have also suggested variations of these 4 predictors as part of a diagnostic algorithm. Singhal and colleagues[12] found that a CRP greater than 20 mg/L was the strongest independent factor. In 2004, Kocher and colleagues[13] completed a validation study of their algorithm, which concluded that its diagnostic performance in a new patient population had diminished. Neither Luhmann and colleagues[14] in 2005 nor Sultan and Hughes[15] in 2010 were able to reproduce the findings of Kocher and colleagues[13] at other institutions. In 2013, Uzoigwe[16] completed a systematic review of previous studies published on diagnostic algorithms. He found that there are significant differences between many of the studies. Furthermore, poor sample size and an insufficient number of actual septic arthritis cases diminishes their reliability. The tendency with such criteria is to depend on them at the exclusion of other very important information, in this case physical examination and, in particular, range of motion. Thus the physician should not depend solely on such algorithms to make the diagnosis. Rather, algorithms should be used as tools in addition to all the information gathered by history, physical examination, and imaging.[6,15–23]

DIAGNOSTIC SUGGESTIONS

The goal of the initial evaluation of a child with hip pain is to try to determine if the cause is septic arthritis. In doing this it is clear that one should not rely on any single piece of information. It is exceedingly important to integrate all data available in making a decision. In this context, however, there are several clinical insights that can be helpful.

First, it is clear that a child not bearing weight would require a referral, but the ability to walk at presentation does not rule out the possibility of a septic hip. Early in the course of sepsis, in partially treated (eg, given oral antibiotics for a sore throat) sepsis, and in immunocompromised patients, walking may be present.

Second, determine if the child looks ill and/or has a fever. There is a definitive difference in the appearance of a child with sepsis and one with transient synovitis or LCP disease.

Third, determine the range of motion and its quality. Pain with flexion and internal rotation is a sensitive indicator of hip irritability/inflammation. It is often the first physical finding present and the last to resolve. Assessment of the range of motion is of particular benefit in differentiating a septic hip from an inflammatory cause. Usually an inflamed hip has pain at the ends of motion. If the hip is moved in the central range of its motion, there is no pain. Pain is elicited when the motion is extended beyond this central arch. A septic hip has pain with all motion.

Fourth, apply the clinical algorithms of Kocher and colleagues[11] and the CRP level[12] in the context of the findings already identified in the aforementioned points.

As a general rule, any painful hip that has motion restriction should be referred. An "ill-looking" child with a fever should probably be referred to the emergency room even if the child is walking. If there is a possibility that there is a septic hip, antibiotics should not be given as part of the referral, regardless of how likely one might think the presence of sepsis might be. Antibiotics can mitigate the physical findings, delay the correct diagnosis, and hinder the growth of cultures.

In cases where septic hip is suspected, an ultrasound-guided hip aspiration can be performed.[8] This aspiration should probably be done at the institution that would definitively drain the septic hip. In borderline cases, admission for observation and bed rest is sometimes indicated. Transient synovitis will usually begin to respond to bed rest within 24 hours. A dose of toradol can often improve the clinical symptoms and shorten the course of transient synovitis substantially.

SUMMARY

The differentiation of septic hip from other inflammatory causes of hip pain in the child can be difficult. In addition, it is essential not to miss or delay the diagnosis of a septic hip. Using knowledge of the presentations of these diagnoses along with good clinical acumen, the physician can achieve these goals. It is important to incorporate all information from the history, physical examination, laboratory tests, and imaging, with an emphasis on range of motion and the judicious use of clinical algorithms. It is certainly better to misdiagnose and treat transient synovitis as a septic hip than to treat a septic hip as a transient synovitis.

REFERENCES

1. Marjolien K, Wouden JC, Schellevis FG, et al. Acute nontraumatic hip pathology in children: incidence and presentation in the family practice. Fam Pract 2010;27: 166–70.
2. Nouri A, Walmsley D, Pruszczynski B, et al. Transient synovitis of the hip: a comprehensive review. J Pediatr Orthop B 2014;23(1):32–6.
3. Kang SN, Sanghera T, Mangwani J, et al. The management of septic arthritis in children: systematic review of the English language literature. J Bone Joint Surg Br 2009;91(9):1127–33.

4. Skaggs DL, Tolo VT. Legg-Calvé-Perthes disease. J Am Acad Orthop Surg 1996; 4:9–16.
5. Seyahi A, Uludag S, Altintas B, et al. Tibial torus and toddler's fracture misdiagnosed as transient synovitis: a case series. J Med Case Rep 2011;5:305.
6. Jung ST, Rowe SM, Moon ES, et al. Significance of laboratory and radiographic findings for differentiating between septic arthritis and transient synovitis of the hip. J Pediatr Orthop 2003;23:368–72.
7. Lee SW, Irwin GJ, Huntley JS. Neonatal hip septic arthritis: ultrasound should not influence decision to aspirate. Scott Med J 2013;58(3):18–21.
8. Zamzam MM. The role of ultrasound in differentiating septic arthritis from transient synovitis of the hip in children. J Pediatr Orthop B 2006;15(6):418–22.
9. Harrison WD, Vooght AK, Singhal R, et al. The epidemiology of transient synovitis in Liverpool, UK. J Child Orthop 2014;8(1):23–8.
10. Kwack KS, Cho JH, Lee JH, et al. Septic arthritis versus transient synovitis of the hip: gadolinium-enhanced MRI finding of decreased perfusion at the femoral epiphysis. AJR Am J Roentgenol 2007;189:437–45.
11. Kocher MS, Zurakowski D, Kasser JR. Differentiation between septic arthritis and transient synovitis of the hip in children: and evidence-based clinical prediction algorithm. J Bone Joint Surg Am 1999;81A:1662–70.
12. Singhal R, Perry DC, Khan FN, et al. The use of CRP within a clinical prediction algorithm for the differentiation of septic arthritis and transient synovitis in children. J Bone Joint Surg Br 2011;93B:1556–61.
13. Kocher MS, Mandiga R, Zurakowski D, et al. Validation of a clinical prediction rule for the differentiation between septic arthritis and transient synovitis of the hip in children. J Bone Joint Surg Am 2004;86:1629–35.
14. Luhmann SJ, Jones A, Schootman M, et al. Differentiation between septic arthritis and transient synovitis of the hip in children with clinical prediction algorithms. J Bone Joint Surg Am 2004;86A(5):956–62.
15. Sultan J, Hughes PJ. Septic arthritis or transient synovitis of the hip: the value of clinical prediction algorithms. J Bone Joint Surg Br 2010;92B(9):1289–93.
16. Uzoigwe CE. Another look: is there a flaw to the current septic arthritis diagnostic algorithms? Clin Orthop Relat Res 2014;472:1645–51.
17. Liberman B, Herman A, Schindler A, et al. The value of hip aspiration in pediatric transient synovitis. J Pediatr Orthop 2013;33:124–7.
18. Eich GF, Superti-Furga A, Umbricht FS, et al. The painful hip: evaluation of criteria for clinical decision-making. Eur J Pediatr 1999;158:923–8.
19. Caird M, Flynn J, Leung Y. Factors distinguishing septic arthritis from transient synovitis of the hip in children. J Bone Joint Surg Am 2006;88A:1251–7.
20. Taekema HC, Landman PR, Maconochie I. Distinguishing between transient synovitis and septic arthritis in the limping child: how useful are clinical prediction tools? Arch Dis Child 2009;94:167–8.
21. Nnadi C, Chawla T, Redfern A, et al. Radiograph evaluation in children with acute hip pain. J Pediatr Orthop 2002;22:342–4.
22. Do TT. Transient synovitis as a cause of painful limps in children. Curr Opin Pediatr 2000;12(1):48–51.
23. Rutz E, Spoerri M. Septic arthritis of the paediatric hip – a review of current diagnostic approaches and therapeutic concepts. Acta Orthop Belg 2013;79(2): 123–34.

Slipped Capital Femoral Epiphysis

How to Evaluate with a Review and Update of Treatment

Andrew G. Georgiadis, MD[a], Ira Zaltz, MD[b]

KEYWORDS

- Slipped capital femoral epiphysis • SCFE • Hip disorders, pediatric • Chondrolysis
- Dunn osteotomy • Osteonecrosis • Avascular necrosis
- Medial circumflex femoral artery

KEY POINTS

- Slipped capital femoral epiphysis (SCFE) is a common adolescent hip disorder.
- The physis is uniquely susceptible to lysis during specific periods of growth, and the risk of epiphyseal displacement is compounded by normal proximal femoral development, physeal orientation, acetabular morphology, and endocrinologic factors.
- Rapid diagnosis can be made by careful clinical history, examination, and performance of anteroposterior and frog-lateral radiographs.

INTRODUCTION

The earliest report of slipped capital femoral epiphysis (SCFE) is widely attributed to a 1572 French text, *Cinq Livres de Chirurgie*, by Ambroise Paré, a barber surgeon for the King of France.[1] Later, Müller described a deformity he termed "bending of the neck of the femur in adolescence."[2] By 1898 there were 22 publications on coxa vara in the German literature alone. The suspected source of deformity in these early studies included fracture,[3] rickettsial disorders,[2] infection,[4] endocrine disturbances, and "periosteal atrophy [. . .] tending to produce a point of weakness at the epiphyseal line."[5]

Sprengel[6] cadaverically proved epiphyseal separation and proposed that SCFE stemmed from fracture. The first etiologic categorization, performed by Key,[5] comprehensively classified proximal femoral varus due to Perthes, infection, Charcot

Disclosure: None.
[a] Department of Orthopaedic Surgery, Henry Ford Hospital, Detroit, MI 48202, USA;
[b] Orthopaedic Surgery, William Beaumont Hospital, 30575 Woodward Avenue, Royal Oak, MI 48073, USA
E-mail address: zaltzira@gmail.com

arthropathy, rickets, congenital deformities, and arthritic causes, with an emphasis on slipped epiphyses. Late nineteenth and early twentieth century investigators differentiated traumatic and insidious proximal femoral epiphyseal separation and suggested early treatment include three or more months of hip spica casting.[3,7] Subtrochanteric cuneiform osteotomies were performed as early as 1900 for a variety of fixed proximal femoral deformities in adolescents, including healed or remodeled SCFE.

PATHOPHYSIOLOGY

The underlying pathologic condition in SCFE involves a mechanical overload to the proximal femoral physis causing anterior translation and external rotation of the metaphysis with respect to the upper femoral epiphysis. At-risk patients are of a characteristic age, with certain epidemiologic, anatomic, histologic, and endocrinologic factors.

Vascular Anatomy

The vascular supply to the proximal femoral epiphysis undergoes series of developmental stages described by Trueta.[8] Before 3 months of age, the developing chondropeiphysis has a significant contribution from the artery of the ligamentum teres, a robust and nearly vertical ascending metaphyseal circulation, and a horizontal precursor to the lateral epiphyseal arteries emanating from the greater trochanter. By 18 months of age, the lateral epiphyseal arteries are the dominant contributors to the femoral head because the ascending metaphyseal arteries no longer cross the physeal plate (**Fig. 1**) and the artery of the ligamentum teres disappears between

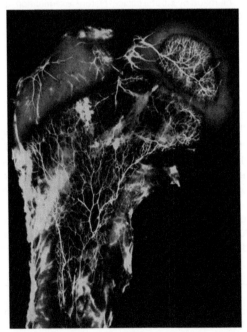

Fig. 1. Specimen from 18-month-old human cadaver. Evident is the complete independence of the lateral epiphyseal arteries investing the epiphysis and the ascending metaphyseal vessels ending at the physeal plate. This independence persists until physeal closure in adolescence. (*From* Trueta J. The normal vascular anatomy of the human femoral head during growth. J Bone Joint Surg Br 1957;39-B(2):358–94; with permission.)

6 months and 3 years of age. Complete independence of the metaphyseal and epiphyseal circulations persists to adulthood. During adolescence and immediately preceding physeal closure, an increasingly rich metaphyseal circulation begins to invest the subphyseal region, ascending to terminate in the hypertrophic zone of the physeal plate (**Fig. 2**) that is the cellular layer through which most SCFE occurs. This metaphyseal supply to the neck arises from the extracapsular arterial ring, distinct from the epiphyseal circulation.

Preceding these experiments, Trueta and Harrison[9] described the intraosseous and extraosseous proximal femoral vascular anatomy in adult hips through a series of detailed histologic dye studies.[9,10] The medial circumflex femoral artery (MFCA) supplies lateral epiphyseal branches that become the dominant vascular contribution to the femoral head by age 18 months and persists into adulthood. The MFCA ascends the posterolateral femoral neck and, once intracapsular, is invested by a fibrous sheath and adjacent venular system.[11] Ganz and colleagues[12] performed detailed dye investigations of the MFCA and lateral epiphyseal vessels, the protection of which can allow for complex surgical exposure of the hip by preservation of the epiphyseal circulation.

Osseous and Physeal Anatomy

Multiple factors differentiate SCFE from a physeal fracture, including antecedent physeolysis, slower displacement, and intact periosteum. Variations in proximal femoral and acetabular anatomy contribute to the pathogenesis of SCFE and physeal instability.

Gelberman and colleagues[13] described relative femoral retroversion in SCFE hips (averaging $1.0°$ vs $6.3°$ of anteversion) and postulated that abnormal torsional stresses, stemming from decreased anteversion, could contribute to rotational instability across the developing growth plate. Later, Sankar and colleagues[14] investigated acetabular anatomy after treatment of unilateral SCFE, demonstrating acetabular retroversion and overcoverage in the unaffected hip, a finding with implications for SCFE development and the development of posttreatment impingement.

The femoral neck-shaft angle decreases from $160°$ at birth to an average of $125°$ degrees by adolescence, along with changes in physeal orientation. Speer[15] described a growth spurt around age 7 resulting in asymmetric neck lengthening and increased verticality of the physis. Mirkopulos and colleagues[16] found that subjects with

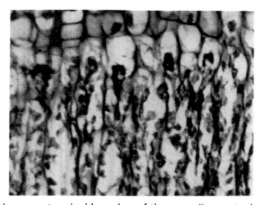

Fig. 2. During adolescence, terminal branches of the ascending metaphyseal circulation do not cross the closing physis, instead they end in the hypertrophic zone of the growth plate. (*From* Trueta J. The normal vascular anatomy of the human femoral head during growth. J Bone Joint Surg Br 1957;39-B(2):358–94; with permission.)

unilateral SCFE had steeper physes than both their unaffected contralateral hips and age-matched controls. A 14° increase in radiographic slope occurred between 1 and 18 years, with the most rapid increase occurring between ages 9 and 12. This higher physeal inclination angle and resultant increase in shear vector parallel to the growth plate may contribute to epiphyseal translation and development of a SCFE.[15,17] Because physiologic loads can create shear forces in excess of six times body weight, obesity further contributes to epiphyseal instability.

The perichondrial ring contributes to the load-carrying capacity of the physeal plate. Because the perichondrial ring thins and attenuates during adolescence, less shear force is necessary to cause epiphyseal displacement.[15,18] Physiologic shear forces have been shown capable of displacing an adolescent proximal femoral epiphysis ex vivo[18,19] furthering the mechanical contribution to SCFE development.

Although the precise pathogenesis is unclear, physeal cellular columnar height and organization are significantly altered in SCFE. Because the perichondrial ring is thinned, the large surface area of the undulating, interlocking mammillary processes provide the greatest internal support of the normal physis. In contrast, SCFE is characterized by physeal widening up to 12 mm (normal range: 2–6 mm), a widened hypertrophic zone comprising 60% to80% of the physeal height, enlargement of chondrocytes, cellular columnar disorganization, higher proteoglycan and extracellular matrix concentrations throughout the physis, and a general disruption in orderly chondrocyte differentiation and endochondral ossification (**Fig. 3**).[15,17,20] Radiographic physeal widening implies a mechanically weakened physis susceptible to unlocking of the mammillary processes and further destabilization.

The epiphyseal tubercle is an anatomic feature receiving increased attention. It is a prominence consistently located among the mammillary processes of the posterosuperior quadrant of the epiphysis.[21] The tubercle averages 4 mm in height, is always below the foramina for the lateral epiphyseal vessels, and is postulated to confer mechanical strength to the physeal plate. It is considered a possible keystone for physeal

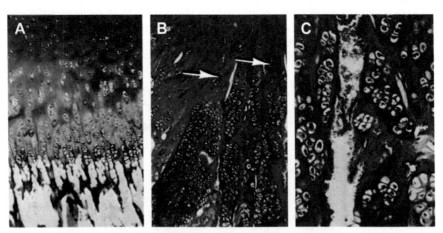

Fig. 3. Normal proximal femoral physis with extracellular matrix primarily in the resting zone and excellent columnar organization of developing chondrocytes (*A*). Proximal femoral physis of an SCFE patient showing extracellular matrix in the proliferating and hypertrophic zones (*B*) and a frank cleft in the hypertrophic zone with disorganized ECM and erythrocytes invasion (*C*). Those *arrows* are demonstrating alcian-blue positivity (proteoglycan content) in the proliferative zone. (*From* Ippolito E, Mickelson MR, Ponseti IV. A histochemical study of slipped capital femoral epiphysis. J Bone Joint Surg Am 1981;63(7):1109–13; with permission.)

stability but decreases in size and surface area during childhood and adolescence as peripheral physeal cupping increases. Liu and colleagues[22] postulate that the epiphysis internally rotates on the epiphyseal tubercle and that a widened physis could contribute to epiphyseal dislodgement. Because the lateral epiphyseal arteries are immediately adjacent to and above the epiphyseal tubercle, this could explain the low rate of osteonecrosis in chronic, stable slips (ie, minimal displacement of the lateral epiphyseal vessels) (**Fig. 4**).

Related Conditions

Suspicion of an endocrinologic disturbance in the pathogenesis of SCFE arose due to the known stippling effect of congenital hypothyroidism because thyroid hormone (T3) is necessary for normal skeletal development and chondrocyte differentiation. Although a common presentation of SCFE is that of an obese, hypogonadal male during the adolescent growth spurt, most SCFEs occur in the absence of endocrine disorder.[23,24]

A stature test can be used to identify patients with SCFE and a concomitant endocrine abnormality.[25] Patients with SCFE who were below the tenth percentile for height comprised 90.9% of all endocrinopathies. Loder and colleagues[26] described the prognostic implications of an age-weight and age-height test to distinguish a typical (idiopathic) from an atypical (usually endocrine-related) SCFE. Subjects were grouped into six categories based on age (<10 years, 10–16 years, >16 years) and weight or height (greater or less than the fiftieth percentile). In combined variable models, extremes of age and weight; height and weight; and age, height, and weight were associated with increased odds-ratios of an atypical slipped epiphysis (**Table 1**). Because these tests all have high negative predictive value, an orthopedic surgeon can be reasonably confident that an SCFE is idiopathic when the age-weight, age-height, and stature tests are negative.

Loder and colleagues[27] published a review of all previously reported slipped capital epiphyses in patients with endocrine disturbances, separating subjects into three groups: hypothyroidism, growth hormone deficiency, and all others. Hypothyroidism was the most common diagnosis (40% of 85 subjects) and the development of SCFE usually antedated the diagnosis of thyroid disturbance. All subjects with growth hormone deficiency (25%) had been diagnosed before developing an SCFE, experienced the shortest symptom duration before a slip diagnosis, and 92% developed

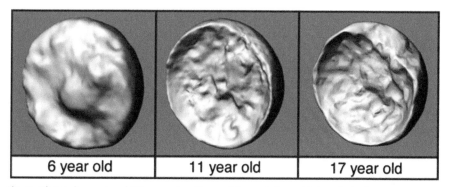

| 6 year old | 11 year old | 17 year old |

Fig. 4. Three dimensional CT reconstructions of the epiphyseal tubercle in the posterosuperior epiphysis, decreasing in normative size as a child ages. Also appreciable is the increase in physeal cupping over time. (*From* Liu RW, Armstrong DG, Levine AD, et al. An anatomic study of the epiphyseal tubercle and its importance in the pathogenesis of slipped capital femoral epiphysis. J Bone Joint Surg Am 2013;95:e341–8; with permission.)

Table 1 Odds ratios of atypical SCFE based on deviations from norms of age, weight, and height	
Group	**Odds Ratio**
Age <10 or >16 y	7.4
Height <50th percentile	6.0
Age and height	
Age <10 or >16 y	5.8
Height <50th percentile	15.0
Weight and height	
Weight <50th percentile	7.4
Height <50th percentile	12.8
Age, weight, and height	
Age <10 or >16 y	4.9
Weight <50th percentile	4.5
Height <50th percentile	14.1

Data from Loder RT, Starnes T, Dikos G. Atypical and typical (idiopathic) slipped capital femoral epiphysis. Reconfirmation of the age-weight test and description of the height and age-height tests. J Bone Joint Surg Am 2006;88(7):1574–81.

a slip during their hormone replacement therapy. All subjects with other endocrine disturbances, such as panhypopituitarism, craniopharyngioma, and multiple endocrine neoplasia (35%), were diagnosed later in adolescence (average age 17.4 years) and an average of 3 years from first SCFE symptoms. Bilaterality is more commonly reported in endocrine-related SCFE,[27,28] with many unilateral presentations progressing to contralateral involvement within the first 18 months. Increased rates of SCFE have also been demonstrated in subjects with renal osteodystrophy and secondary hyperparathyroidism,[29] postradiation,[30] hypogonadism,[31] and Down syndrome.[32]

A unique combination of histologic, vascular, anatomic, and endocrinologic factors affect physeal stability and the pathogenesis of SCFE. The proximal femoral physis represents an area of rapid cellular proliferation vulnerable to instability, is characterized by a unique temporal susceptibility that can be heightened by the body's endocrinologic milieu, and is nourished by a fragile blood supply.

CLINICAL EVALUATION

Patients with slipped capital epiphyses can present to a physician in a delayed or acute fashion with implications for epiphyseal stability. Patients commonly present with longstanding symptoms lasting months. The most common presentations include limp and pain in the affected groin, lateral or posterior hip, thigh, or ipsilateral knee. Knee pain in SCFE is referred by a reflex arc involving somatic sensory nerves ending at the same spinal level (**Fig. 5**). This differs from radiating pain caused by irritation of obturator nerve branches that course to the medial knee. Knee pain, present in 15% to 50% of SCFE, leads to high rates of misdiagnosis, extra radiographs, higher grade SCFE at treatment,[33,34] and errant surgical procedures directed at nonexistent knee disease.[35] A stable slip, Medicaid insurance, and distal thigh or knee pain are the strongest independent predictors of a delay in diagnosis of SCFE.[34]

Altered gait patterns in SCFE include components of antalgic, waddling, or Trendelenburg gait, with an externally rotated foot progression angle. Only a small

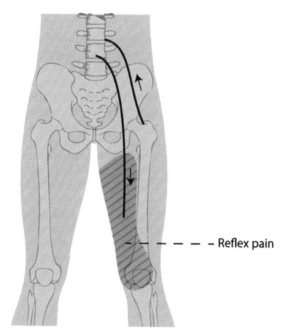

Fig. 5. Reflex arc of referred pain in SCFE, in which a reflex of afferent somatic sensory nerves from the hip terminate at a spinal level in proximity to efferent pain signals to the knee and thigh.

percentage of limp in SCFE is painless.[36] Motion can be severely restricted in multiple planes and rotational profiles should be compared bilaterally. Patients may have weak hip abduction, decreased hip flexion, decreased internal rotation, obligate external rotation with hip flexion (Drehmann sign), and the development of synovitis precipitating a flexed posture or even hip flexion contracture. A positive Drehmann sign is elicited when the examiner passive flexes the supine patient's hip, which then falls into obligate external rotation and abduction.[37]

Reviews of large national databases report an SCFE incidence rate of 10 per 100,000, with a 1.4:2.0 female/male ratio. The average age of diagnosis is 12 years, and most patients presenting outside of ages 10 and 16 represent atypical SCFE possibly associated with endocrinologic diagnoses.[26] Blacks, Hispanics, and Pacific Islanders have significantly greater incidence rates than whites. There has been a consistent finding of higher SCFE incidence north of 40° latitude, with the greatest incidences in the United States found in the Northeast and West. A seasonal incidence pattern has also been noted, with most northern latitudes presenting in the summer months, and most southern latitudes in the winter.[38,39] Recent data have indicated a trend to decreased age and increased frequency of bilaterality at first presentation, suspected to correlate with increasing rates of childhood obesity.[40]

Bilateral SCFE at first presentation has traditionally been reported in approximately 20%, with higher rates in patients with endocrinopathy.[25,26] The incidence of metachronous slip, affecting 15% to 36% of SCFE, may provide justification for prophylactic pinning of the unaffected hip in at-risk patients.[41,42] Almost 90% of metachronous SCFE presents within the first 18 months after treatment of the index slip.[43]

RADIOGRAPHIC EVALUATION

The primary radiographic test used in suspected SCFE remains an anteroposterior (AP) and frog pelvis radiograph. Klein and colleagues[44] described a line drawn along the superior neck on the AP image that should intersect the epiphysis. Failure to do so comprises a positive Trethowan sign and may indicate a slipped femoral epiphysis. The sensitivity of this line has been questioned, reportedly missing 61% of SCFE and underdiagnosing patients in a preslip phase.[45] Green and colleagues[46] found similarly low sensitivity of this line, proposing a modification wherein the amount of the epiphysis that is lateral to the Klein line was compared between the two hips on the AP image, with a 2 mm side-to-side difference highly suspicious of SCFE. There are numerous subtle radiographic findings indicating early slippage, including widening and irregularity of the affected physis, sharpening of the metaphyseal border of the head, loss of anterior concavity to the head-neck junction on the lateral view, and subtle periosteal elevation[44,47]; however, lateral radiographs are generally more sensitive than the AP images, particularly in the earliest phases of slipping (**Fig. 6**). Most SCFE is characterized by anterior translation and external rotation of the metaphysis relative to the epiphysis, which, on an AP projection, is located posterior and inferior to the metaphysis. As a result, the total epiphyseal height may appear decreased and a double-density or metaphyseal blanch sign described by Steel[48] can be present. Chronic SCFE can result in uncovering and resorption of the superior metaphysis, with periosteal reaction, osseous formation, and breaking along the inferomedial neck (**Fig. 7**).

The role of advanced imaging is controversial and generally used on a case-by-case basis. Ultrasound can detect the presence of hip effusion and a step-off at the epiphyseal-metaphyseal junction.[49] CT allows for the assessment of physeal closure or morphologic assessment of proximal femoral deformity, particularly with three-dimensional reconstruction if complex osteotomy is planned. Intraarticular hardware penetration is also best assessed by CT.[50] MRI can assess vascularity to the femoral head or the extent of AVN.

CLASSIFICATION

Symptom duration has been used to classify SCFE as acute, chronic, or acute-on-chronic. Acute SCFE comprises 10% to 15% of all SCFE, and presents within 3 weeks

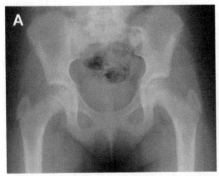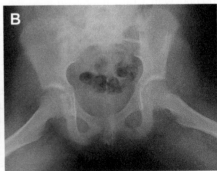

Fig. 6. AP and lateral radiographs of a right slipped capital epiphysis in a 10-year old female. (A) On the AP projection, the Klein's line intersects both epiphyses. A modified Klein's line would reveal asymmetry in the quantity of epiphysis intersected. The right physis is obviously widened compared to the unaffected left. (B) A frog lateral projection reveals posterior slippage and loss of anterior convexity of the head-neck junction.

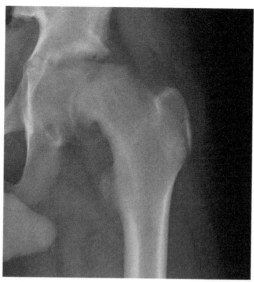

Fig. 7. AP hip radiographic demonstrating chronic remodeling in chronic SCFE. There is periosteal reaction and breaking along the inferior neck, and rounding and blunting of the superior metaphysis due to resorption.

of the onset of symptoms. Acute presentation is associated with a higher rate of avascular necrosis (AVN)[51] and can present after trauma or an identifiable inciting injury. Chronic SCFE, comprising 85% of cases, implies at least 3 weeks of symptoms. Patients with prodromal symptoms of pain and limp have been known to experience a new injury with immediate worsening, a so-called acute-on-chronic slip.[11] Temporal classification is useful for describing chronicity but has less prognostic value.

Loder and colleagues[43] introduced the concept of physeal stability, categorizing SCFE as either stable or unstable based on the subject's ability to bear weight, even with crutches. Physeal stability was predictive of osteonecrosis rates, with 47% of unstable and 0% of stable slips developing AVN within 6 to 18 months. There is marked heterogeneity in the application of the stable or unstable classification in the literature.[52] More recently analyzed historical data suggest the rate of osteonecrosis in unstable SCFE is closer to 23.9%.[53]

Radiographic severity grading was described by epiphyseal displacement as a fraction of total physeal diameter.[47,54] By this grading, slips can be mild (<33%), moderate (33%–50%), or severe (>50%). A more commonly used classification is the slip angle of Southwick[55] in which the difference in the angle subtended by the proximal femoral physis and the ipsilateral femoral shaft are compared between affected and unaffected sides. Differences less than 30° are mild, between 30 and 50° are moderate, and greater than 50° are severe. Because femoral rotation can vary depending on radiographic technique and patient comfort, the Southwick grading is inconsistent.[56]

TREATMENT

SCFE requires surgical management, except in rare instances, because stabilization of the epiphysis and early fusion of the proximal femoral physis prevents further displacement and deformity. The preferred treatment of SCFE has undergone dramatic change as surgical techniques have evolved and imaging has improved. There remains considerable debate about the optimal treatment of stable SCFE. Recommendations will be refined if long-term, prospective data becomes available and as surgeons are trained in increasingly complex hip surgery.

Closed Reduction and Spica Casting

Deliberate manipulation and closed reduction of a slipped epiphysis is largely historical. Some investigators have reported low rates of osteonecrosis if gentle, deliberate manipulation was performed within 24 hours of presentation, presumably because contracture and shortening of the ascending cervical branches of the MFCA had yet to occur.[57] Spontaneous reduction refers to a nondeliberate change in metaphyseal-epiphyseal relationships that usually occurs during patient positioning on a surgical table immediately preceding treatment. Spontaneous reduction has been reported to occur in up to 90% of unstable and 8% of stable slips.[43,52]

Casting as a sole treatment modality or in conjunction with closed reduction was almost entirely abandoned in the developed world by the late 1950s. Historically, patients were immobilized in a position of extension, abduction, and external rotation. Many series have reported high rates of slip progression, chondrolysis, pressure ulcers,[3,7] and recurrence of slip even up to 11 months after recumbent spica immobilization.[47] Long-term Swedish data with an average of 46-year follow-up revealed a harmful influence of both closed reduction and hip spica casting when compared with symptomatic or no treatment.[58] Reduction and hip spica casting resulted in higher rates of subsequent hip surgery and more late arthrosis.

Open Reduction and Physiodesis

The primary goal of SCFE treatment is stabilization and arrest of the proximal femoral physis. Historically, the rates of physiodesis with the earliest, large metallic implants (Smith-Peterson nails, Hagie pins) were unsatisfactory; therefore, Heyman and Herndon[59] described manipulative reduction and bone peg epiphysiodesis. Their subjects experienced rapid fusion of the proximal femoral physis (2.3 months), much shorter than classic conservative treatment. Comparably good functional series with open epiphysiodesis were reproduced for decades thereafter.[11] A fundamental drawback to the procedure was a larger and more morbid anterior exposure; subsequently, it became less popular as screw fixation methods improved.

In Situ Fixation

In situ screw fixation to prevent further epiphyseal displacement and to induce physeal arrest is currently the most common treatment of SCFE of all types (stable or unstable), regardless of degree of deformity.[52] Correct insertion requires placing the screw perpendicular to the epiphysis, crossing the physis into the geometric center of the femoral head.[60] With increasing slip displacement, the epiphysis location is more posterior relative to the femoral neck, requiring a more anterior starting point on the neck to cross perpendicularly into the epiphysis (**Fig. 8**). Percutaneous fixation was accomplished exclusively with solid or threaded pins until the introduction of cannulated screws. There are many current variations in placement technique.[61]

Percutaneous in situ fixation can be performed either by positioning the patient supine on a radiolucent operating table or on a fracture table. Most surgeons use cannulated screws to increase the chances of center-center fixation.[62] There is no proven biomechanical or clinical advantage to the use of multiple screws versus a single screw.[60,63] Liu and colleagues[22] suggest that single in situ screw fixation should not be placed in the posterosuperior quadrant of the femoral head, the location of

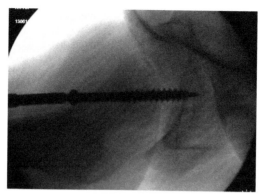

Fig. 8. An intraoperative fluoroscopic image of a moderate slip with relative posterior epiphyseal displacement. This necessitates an anterior starting point at the base of the femoral neck across the physis perpendicularly and engaging center-center in the head.

the epiphyseal tubercle, because the epiphysis could theoretically pivot around this single, fixed point.

The most important technical considerations during percutaneous in situ fixation are center-center fixation within the epiphysis and avoiding intraarticular penetration. Walters and Simon[64] geometrically detailed the manner by which joint penetration could be overlooked, even with seemingly intraosseous metallic pins on AP, lateral, and frog-lateral images. They described a safe-zone for placement when static images are obtained. Despite exacting radiographic techniques, Senthi and colleagues[50] demonstrated that screws terminating closer than 4 mm to the subchondral bone on lateral images may penetrate the joint. Other methods, including injection of dye into a cannulated screw, were developed to mitigate risk of screw penetration and development of chondrolysis.[65]

Prophylactic pinning of a radiographically and clinically normal hip is generally reserved for patients with nonidiopathic SCFE (ie, <10 or >16 years of age), SCFE associated with endocrinopathy, or in obese patients with delayed presentation in whom the surgeon suspects a delay would ensue in the presentation of metachronous SCFE. Historically, even in the case of unilateral SCFE in a patient with endocrinopathy, wherein the metachronous slip rate is 70%, routine prophylactic pinning of the asymptomatic hip has been contested.[25] Currently, there is a growing body of evidence that supports routine prophylactic in situ fixation in unilateral SCFE because the associated complication rate is acceptable compared with the high incidence of complications from a contralateral SCFE.[66–68]

Contemporary Surgical Treatments

Modern open surgery for treatment of SCFE can be technically challenging and its role remains controversial. Unsatisfactory clinical results reported in 10% to 20% of patients treated with in situ pin fixation has lead some to advocate that, for severe deformities, surgeons should attempt to downgrade the degree of deformity or to correct the deformity to mitigate the long-term risk of cartilage damage.[69–72] For mild SCFE or healed proximal femoral deformity producing impingement, surgical dislocation, limited anterior open or arthroscopic approaches with femoral neck osteochondroplasty have been reported.[73–75]

Osteotomy can be performed at the intertrochanteric, basicervical, or subcapital levels depending on the extent of physeal healing and degree of deformity. Goals of this treatment include redirection of the femoral head to minimize femoroacetabular impingement and to improve functional range of motion. Contracture of the posterior retinacular vessels occurs in the setting of a chronic slip, necessitating femoral neck shortening to avoid tension causing occlusion and AVN if a head or neck osteotomy is to be performed (**Fig. 9**). The modified Dunn procedure, an intracapsular wedge

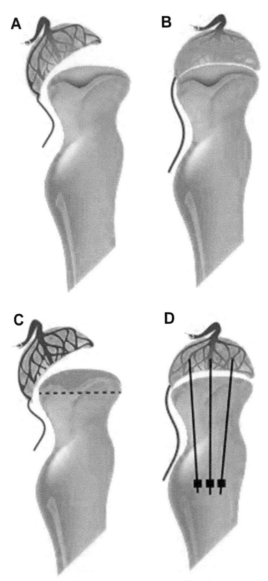

Fig. 9. In chronic SCFE, the posterior vessels are shortened and contracted (*A*) and acute reduction results in high rates of AVN (*B*). A functional shortening and relaxation of the epiphyseal vasculature can be achieved with a cuneiform neck osteotomy (*C*) preceding epiphyseal reduction (*D*). (*Adapted from* Dunn DM. The treatment of adolescent slipping of the upper femoral epiphysis. J Bone Joint Surg Br 1964;46:621–9.)

osteotomy of the femoral neck with reduction of the head, has been reported in the treatment of unstable SCFE with short-term results.[76–79]

Loder and Dietz[52] suggest that a surgical dislocation approach has insufficient evidence in either stable or unstable situations, citing an increased rate of AVN using surgical dislocation or modified Dunn as a treatment of stable SCFE (7% vs 0%). They recommend that select centers undertake a prospective evaluation of surgical dislocation and modified Dunn osteotomy, cautioning against its routine use.

COMPLICATIONS

All treatments of SCFE share the common goals of epiphyseal stabilization and preventing serious complications, including chondrolysis and osteonecrosis of the femoral epiphysis. Loder and colleagues[43] original description of physeal stability reported 0% AVN in stable and 47% in unstable slips. Recently reported composite rates from 15 clinical studies places the osteonecrosis rate of unstable slips at 23.9%.[53] It remains controversial whether acute reduction contributes to or could improve vascularity of the epiphysis because superselective angiography of the superior retinacular vessels has shown restoration of epiphyseal flow after acute reduction of the epiphysis.[80]

Chondrolysis, a loss of the cartilaginous surface of the femoral head and acetabulum, has been reported following all methods of treatment of SCFE. Patients present with global loss of motion and pain. Radiographically, the diagnosis is suspected when there is loss of compared joint space and osteopenia. The highest rates occur following nonoperative treatment,[81] especially high-grade slips,[54] and in 1.5% of patients treated with percutaneous in situ fixation.[82] Chondrolysis can occur with or without evidence of guide wire or implant penetration during or following surgery, though most investigators recommend avoiding intraarticular penetration regardless of its causative role.[83] Anterior femoroacetabular impingement as a result of residual femoral metaphyseal prominence has been implicated in late-presenting chondrolysis.[84]

Recurrence or progression of a slipped epiphysis has been reported even after prolonged spica cast treatment[47] and other modes of stabilization.[85] It is more likely to occur in nonidiopathic SCFE or following in situ stabilization of severe deformities. The true prevalence of this complication is not known with specificity.

SUMMARY

SCFE is a common adolescent hip disorder. The physis is uniquely susceptible to lysis during specific periods of growth and the risk of epiphyseal displacement is compounded by normal proximal femoral development, physeal orientation, acetabular morphology, and endocrinologic factors. It is most clinically useful to classify SCFE by physeal stability, determined by the patient's ability to bear weight. Rapid diagnosis can be made by careful clinical history, examination, and performance of AP and frog-lateral radiographs. Single in situ screw fixation across the physis predictably stabilizes the epiphysis and accelerates physeal closure. There is increasing use of open reduction, especially following acute SCFE and reconstruction for symptomatic chronic SCFE, though the precise role for these procedures is not yet defined.

REFERENCES

1. Paré A. Cinq livres de chirurgie. Wechel; 1572.
2. Müller E. The classic: 1 on the deflection of the femoral neck in childhood a new syndrome. Clin Orthop Relat Res 1966;48:7–10.

3. Whitman RI. Further observations on depression of the neck of the femur in early life; including fracture of the neck of the femur, separation of the epiphysis and simple coxa vara. Ann Surg 1900;31:145–62.

4. Frohelich. Ztschr f orthop chir. 1904;12:80.

5. Key JA. Epiphyseal coxa vara or displacement of the capital epiphysis of the femur in adolescence. J Bone Joint Surg 1926;8:53–117.

6. Sprengel Arch f klin Chir. 1898;57:805.

7. Wilson PD. Displacement of upper epiphysis of femur treated by open reduction. J Am Med Assoc 1924;83:1749–56.

8. Trueta J. The normal vascular anatomy of the human femoral head during growth. J Bone Joint Surg Br 1957;39-B:358–94.

9. Trueta J, Harrison MH. The normal vascular anatomy of the femoral head in adult man. J Bone Joint Surg Br 1953;35-B:442–61.

10. Wertheimer LG, Lopes Sde L. Arterial supply of the femoral head. A combined angiographic and histological study. J Bone Joint Surg Am 1971;53:545–56.

11. Aadalen RJ, Weiner DS, Hoyt W, et al. Acute slipped capital femoral epiphysis. J Bone Joint Surg Am 1974;56:1473–87.

12. Gautier E, Ganz K, Krugel N, et al. Anatomy of the medial femoral circumflex artery and its surgical implications. J Bone Joint Surg Br 2000;82:679–83.

13. Gelberman RH, Cohen MS, Shaw BA, et al. The association of femoral retroversion with slipped capital femoral epiphysis. J Bone Joint Surg Am 1986;68:1000–7.

14. Sankar WN, Brighton BK, Kim YJ, et al. Acetabular morphology in slipped capital femoral epiphysis. J Pediatr Orthop 2011;31:254–8.

15. Speer DP. The John Charnley Award Paper. Experimental epiphysiolysis: etiologic models slipped capital femoral epiphysis. Hip 1982;68–88.

16. Mirkopulos N, Weiner DS, Askew M. The evolving slope of the proximal femoral growth plate relationship to slipped capital femoral epiphysis. J Pediatr Orthop 1988;8:268–73.

17. Ippolito E, Mickelson MR, Ponseti IV. A histochemical study of slipped capital femoral epiphysis. J Bone Joint Surg Am 1981;63:1109–13.

18. Chung SM, Batterman SC, Brighton CT. Shear strength of the human femoral capital epiphyseal plate. J Bone Joint Surg Am 1976;58:94–103.

19. Litchman HM, Duffy J. Slipped capital femoral epiphysis: factors affecting shear forces on the epiphyseal plate. J Pediatr Orthop 1984;4:745–8.

20. Ponseti IV, McClintock R. The pathology of slipping of the upper femoral epiphysis. J Bone Joint Surg Am 1956;38-A:71–83.

21. Tayton K. Does the upper femoral epiphysis slip or rotate? J Bone Joint Surg Br 2007;89:1402–6.

22. Liu RW, Armstrong DG, Levine AD, et al. An anatomic study of the epiphyseal tubercle and its importance in the pathogenesis of slipped capital femoral epiphysis. J Bone Joint Surg Am 2013;95:e341–8.

23. Razzano CD, Nelson C, Eversman J. Growth hormone levels in slipped capital femoral epiphysis. J Bone Joint Surg Am 1972;54:1224–6.

24. Mann DC, Weddington J, Richton S. Hormonal studies in patients with slipped capital femoral epiphysis without evidence of endocrinopathy. J Pediatr Orthop 1988;8:543–5.

25. Burrow SR, Alman B, Wright JG. Short stature as a screening test for endocrinopathy in slipped capital femoral epiphysis. J Bone Joint Surg Br 2001;83:263–8.

26. Loder RT, Starnes T, Dikos G. Atypical and typical (idiopathic) slipped capital femoral epiphysis. Reconfirmation of the age-weight test and description of the height and age-height tests. J Bone Joint Surg Am 2006;88:1574–81.

27. Loder RT, Wittenberg B, DeSilva G. Slipped capital femoral epiphysis associated with endocrine disorders. J Pediatr Orthop 1995;15:349–56.
28. Wells D, King JD, Roe TF, et al. Review of slipped capital femoral epiphysis associated with endocrine disease. J Pediatr Orthop 1993;13:610–4.
29. Loder RT, Hensinger RN. Slipped capital femoral epiphysis associated with renal failure osteodystrophy. J Pediatr Orthop 1997;17:205–11.
30. Wolf EL, Berdon WE, Cassady JR, et al. Slipped femoral capital epiphysis as a sequela to childhood irradiation for malignant tumors. Radiology 1977;125: 781–4.
31. Hirsch PJ, Hirsch SA. Slipped capital femoral epiphysis. Occurrence after treatment with chorionic gonadotropin. JAMA 1976;235:751.
32. Stack RE, Peterson LF. Slipped capital femoral epiphysis and Down's disease. Clin Orthop Relat Res 1966;48:111–7.
33. Matava MJ, Patton CM, Luhmann S, et al. Knee pain as the initial symptom of slipped capital femoral epiphysis: an analysis of initial presentation and treatment. J Pediatr Orthop 1999;19:455–60.
34. Kocher MS, Bishop JA, Weed B, et al. Delay in diagnosis of slipped capital femoral epiphysis. Pediatrics 2004;113:e322–5.
35. Kaplan SR, Klinghoffer L. Knee pain in slipped femoral capital epiphysis causing a delay in diagnosis. Am J Surg 1961;101:798–802.
36. Cowell HR. The significance of early diagnosis and treatment of slipping of the capital femoral epiphysis. Clin Orthop Relat Res 1966;48:89–94.
37. Drehmann F. Drehmann's sign. A clinical examination method in epiphysiolysis (slipping of the upper femoral epiphysis). Description of signs, aetiopathogenetic considerations, clinical experience (author's transl). Z Orthop Ihre Grenzgeb 1979;117:333–44 [in German].
38. Loder RT. The demographics of slipped capital femoral epiphysis. An international multicenter study. Clin Orthop Relat Res 1996;(322):8–27.
39. Lehmann CL, Arons RR, Loder RT, et al. The epidemiology of slipped capital femoral epiphysis: an update. J Pediatr Orthop 2006;26:286–90.
40. Nasreddine AY, Heyworth BE, Zurakowski D, et al. A reduction in body mass index lowers risk for bilateral slipped capital femoral epiphysis. Clin Orthop Relat Res 2013;471(7):2137–44.
41. Hurley JM, Betz RR, Loder RT, et al. Slipped capital femoral epiphysis. The prevalence of late contralateral slip. J Bone Joint Surg Am 1996;78:226–30.
42. Baghdadi YM, Larson AN, Sierra RJ, et al. The fate of hips that are not prophylactically pinned after unilateral slipped capital femoral epiphysis. Clin Orthop Relat Res 2013;471(7):2124–31.
43. Loder RT, Richards BS, Shapiro PS, et al. Acute slipped capital femoral epiphysis: the importance of physeal stability. J Bone Joint Surg Am 1993;75: 1134–40.
44. Klein A, Joplin RJ, Reidy JA, et al. Roentgenographic features of slipped capital femoral epiphysis. Am J Roentgenol Radium Ther 1951;66:361–74.
45. Pinkowsky GJ, Hennrikus WL. Klein line on the anteroposterior radiograph is not a sensitive diagnostic radiologic test for slipped capital femoral epiphysis. J Pediatr 2013;162:804–7.
46. Green DW, Mogekwu N, Scher DM, et al. A modification of Klein's Line to improve sensitivity of the anterior-posterior radiograph in slipped capital femoral epiphysis. J Pediatr Orthop 2009;29:449–53.
47. Wilson PD. The treatment of slipping of the upper femoral epiphysis with minimal displacement. J Bone Joint Surg 1938;20:379–99.

48. Steel HH. The metaphyseal blanch sign of slipped capital femoral epiphysis. J Bone Joint Surg Am 1986;68:920–2.
49. Kallio PE, Paterson DC, Foster BK, et al. Classification in slipped capital femoral epiphysis. Sonographic assessment of stability and remodeling. Clin Orthop Relat Res 1993;(294):196–203.
50. Senthi S, Blyth P, Metcalfe R, et al. Screw placement after pinning of slipped capital femoral epiphysis: a postoperative CT scan study. J Pediatr Orthop 2011;31:388–92.
51. Aronsson DD, Loder RT. Treatment of the unstable (acute) slipped capital femoral epiphysis. Clin Orthop Relat Res 1996;(322):99–110.
52. Loder RT, Dietz FR. What is the best evidence for the treatment of slipped capital femoral epiphysis? J Pediatr Orthop 2012;32(Suppl 2):S158–65.
53. Zaltz I, Baca G, Clohisy JC. Unstable SCFE: review of treatment modalities and prevalence of osteonecrosis. Clin Orthop Relat Res 2013;471(7):2192–8.
54. Wilson PD, Jacobs B, Schecter L. Slipped capital femoral epiphysis: an end-result study. J Bone Joint Surg Am 1965;47:1128–45.
55. Southwick WO. Osteotomy through the lesser trochanter for slipped capital femoral epiphysis. J Bone Joint Surg Am 1967;49:807–35.
56. Loder RT. Effect of femur position on the angular measurement of slipped capital femoral epiphysis. J Pediatr Orthop 2001;21:488–94.
57. Peterson MD, Weiner DS, Green NE, et al. Acute slipped capital femoral epiphysis: the value and safety of urgent manipulative reduction. J Pediatr Orthop 1997;17:648–54.
58. Ordeberg G, Hansson LI, Sandstrom S. Slipped capital femoral epiphysis in southern Sweden. Long-term result with closed reduction and hip plaster spica. Clin Orthop Relat Res 1987;(220):148–54.
59. Heyman CH, Herndon CH. Epiphy seodesis for early slipping of the upper femoral epiphysis. J Bone Joint Surg Am 1954;36-A:539–55.
60. Kibiloski LJ, Doane RM, Karol LA, et al. Biomechanical analysis of single- versus double-screw fixation in slipped capital femoral epiphysis at physiological load levels. J Pediatr Orthop 1994;14:627–30.
61. Gourineni P. Oblique in situ screw fixation of stable slipped capital femoral epiphysis. J Pediatr Orthop 2013;33:135–8.
62. Aronson DD, Loder RT. Slipped capital femoral epiphysis in black children. J Pediatr Orthop 1992;12:74–9.
63. Karol LA, Doane RM, Cornicelli SF, et al. Single versus double screw fixation for treatment of slipped capital femoral epiphysis: a biomechanical analysis. J Pediatr Orthop 1992;12:741–5.
64. Walters R, Simon SR. Joint destruction: a sequel of unrecognized pin penetration in patients with SCFE, The Hip: Proceedings of the 8th Open Scientific Meeting of the Hip Society. St. Louis (MO); 1980. p. 145–64.
65. Lehman WB, Grant A, Rose D, et al. A method of evaluating possible pin penetration in slipped capital femoral epiphysis using a cannulated internal fixation device. Clin Orthop Relat Res 1984;(186):65–70.
66. Seller K, Raab P, Wild A, et al. Risk-benefit analysis of prophylactic pinning in slipped capital femoral epiphysis. J Pediatr Orthop B 2001;10:192–6.
67. Woelfle JV, Fraitzl CR, Reichel H, et al. The asymptomatic contralateral hip in unilateral slipped capital femoral epiphysis: morbidity of prophylactic fixation. J Pediatr Orthop B 2012;21:226–9.
68. Sankar WN, Novais EN, Lee C, et al. What are the risks of prophylactic pinning to prevent contralateral slipped capital femoral epiphysis? Clin Orthop Relat Res 2013;471:2118–23.

69. Millis MB, Zaltz I. Emerging concepts in slipped capital femoral epiphysis: editorial comment. Clin Orthop Relat Res 2013;471(7):2083–4.
70. Witbreuk MM, Bolkenbaas M, Mullender MG, et al. The results of downgrading moderate and severe slipped capital femoral epiphysis by an early Imhauser femur osteotomy. J Child Orthop 2009;3:405–10.
71. Sink EL, Zaltz I, Heare T, et al. Acetabular cartilage and labral damage observed during surgical hip dislocation for stable slipped capital femoral epiphysis. J Pediatr Orthop 2010;30:26–30.
72. Lee CB, Matheney T, Yen YM. Case reports: acetabular damage after mild slipped capital femoral epiphysis. Clin Orthop Relat Res 2013;471:2163–72.
73. Clohisy JC, Zebala LP, Nepple JJ, et al. Combined hip arthroscopy and limited open osteochondroplasty for anterior femoroacetabular impingement. J Bone Joint Surg Am 2010;92:1697–706.
74. Leunig M, Horowitz K, Manner H, et al. In situ pinning with arthroscopic osteoplasty for mild SCFE: a preliminary technical report. Clin Orthop Relat Res 2010; 468:3160–7.
75. Leunig M, Slongo T, Kleinschmidt M, et al. Subcapital correction osteotomy in slipped capital femoral epiphysis by means of surgical hip dislocation. Oper Orthop Traumatol 2007;19:389–410.
76. Ziebarth K, Zilkens C, Spencer S, et al. Capital realignment for moderate and severe SCFE using a modified Dunn procedure. Clin Orthop Relat Res 2009; 467:704–16.
77. Sankar WN, Vanderhave KL, Matheney T, et al. The modified Dunn procedure for unstable slipped capital femoral epiphysis: a multicenter perspective. J Bone Joint Surg Am 2013;95:585–91.
78. Slongo T, Kakaty D, Krause F, et al. Treatment of slipped capital femoral epiphysis with a modified Dunn procedure. J Bone Joint Surg Am 2010;92:2898–908.
79. Huber H, Dora C, Ramseier LE, et al. Adolescent slipped capital femoral epiphysis treated by a modified Dunn osteotomy with surgical hip dislocation. J Bone Joint Surg Br 2011;93:833–8.
80. Maeda S, Kita A, Funayama K, et al. Vascular supply to slipped capital femoral epiphysis. J Pediatr Orthop 2001;21:664–7.
81. Waldenstrom H. On necrosis of the joint cartilage by epiphyseolysis capitis femoris. 1930. Clin Orthop Relat Res 1996;(322):3–7.
82. Kennedy JP, Weiner DS. Results of slipped capital femoral epiphysis in the black population. J Pediatr Orthop 1990;10:224–7.
83. Rooks MD, Schmitt EW, Drvaric DM. Unrecognized pin penetration in slipped capital femoral epiphysis. Clin Orthop Relat Res 1988;(234):82–9.
84. Leunig M, Casillas MM, Hamlet M, et al. Slipped capital femoral epiphysis: early mechanical damage to the acetabular cartilage by a prominent femoral metaphysis. Acta Orthop Scand 2000;71:370–5.
85. Boyer DW, Mickelson MR, Ponseti IV. Slipped capital femoral epiphysis. Long-term follow-up study of one hundred and twenty-one patients. J Bone Joint Surg Am 1981;63:85–95.

Assessment and Treatment of Hip Pain in the Adolescent Athlete

Brian D. Giordano, MD

KEYWORDS

- Hip • Pain • Adolescent • Sports • Groin • Femoroacetabular impingement
- Physeal injury • Acetabular labrum

KEY POINTS

- A thorough history can often uncover important clues about the etiology of pain, and a well-directed interview is crucial to understanding primary versus secondary pain generators in the hip and pelvis.
- The clinician treating hip pain in the adolescent athlete should become familiar with performing a thorough hip examination and interpreting radiographic images. The physician should recognize that a comprehensive hip examination includes evaluation of gait, the spine, abdominovisceral structures, and other musculoskeletal regions.
- Hip pain in the adolescent athlete often reflects a number of concomitant pathologies, and a thorough awareness of the distinct characteristics of each is important to establishing a proper diagnosis and treatment strategy.
- Biomechanical relationships between the hip joint, periarticular soft tissue envelope, and central pelvic structures must be understood to distinguish between primary pathologies and compensatory injury patterns.
- Underlying systemic, rheumatologic, or oncologic conditions should always be considered in the young athlete, even when the injury seems to reflect a musculoskeletal etiology.

 A video of Impingement and instability testing accompanies this article at http://www.pediatric.theclinics.com/

INTRODUCTION

Establishing an accurate diagnosis for the adolescent athlete with hip pain can be challenging. Complex pathomechanical interactions within the hip joint,

Disclosures: Educational and research support: Arthrex, Carticept, Exactech, Smith and Nephew; Consultant: Arthrex, Carticept; Royalties/Stock: None.
Division of Sports Medicine, Department of Orthopaedics, University of Rochester, Box 665, 601 Elmwood Avenue, Rochester, NY 14642, USA
E-mail address: Brian_giordano@urmc.rochester.edu

pediatric.theclinics.com

compensatory extra-articular injuries, and the central watershed location of the hip often result in an obscure clinical picture without a clear singular diagnosis. Open physes among athletes of this age group are prone to overuse enthesopathies, or traumatic avulsions in higher-energy injuries. Morphologic alterations in the proximal femur or acetabulum can result in anatomic conflict during dynamic activities, and may result in debilitating chondral and labral injuries as a young athlete develops. In addition to physeal injuries and femoroacetabular impingement, repetitive microtrauma, or isolated traumatic events can lead to a number of other soft tissue and bony abnormalities that may contribute to hip pain.

HISTORY

An accurate diagnosis for an adolescent athlete with hip pain can usually be gained through a focused clinical history. Of primary concern is whether the onset of symptoms was acute and caused by a single traumatic event, related to repetitive athletic activities, or unrelated to athletic endeavors altogether. Higher-energy athletic injuries to the hip and pelvis frequently involve the biomechanically vulnerable physes and surrounding soft tissues, rather than deeper intra-articular structures. Young elite-level athletes are under increasing pressure to commit to a single sport at a young age, and train throughout the year to optimize their performance in that sport. The literature is replete with the unfortunate consequences of multiple exposure hours to the skeletally immature athlete.[1] Attritional injuries to the acetabular labrum or articular cartilage, stress reactions/fractures, and injuries to the surrounding myotendinous envelope are injury patterns that are linked to repetitive overuse. Fluctuations of symptoms with a diurnal pattern may reflect an underlying inflammatory, systemic, or rheumatologic condition. Pain that is not reproducible with strenuous activities, is not reported with a predictable pattern, and is associated with other vague constitutional symptoms should prompt concern for an underlying systemic etiology (**Figs. 1** and **2**). Inquiring about age at symptomatic onset and development of secondary sex characteristics can yield valuable information about the state of skeletal maturity and certain age-specific cues that may aid in making an accurate diagnosis. Legg Calve Perthes (LCP) and slipped capital femoral epiphysis (SCFE) are 2 conditions that have characteristic age associations and may demonstrate many clinical features similar to

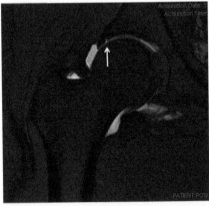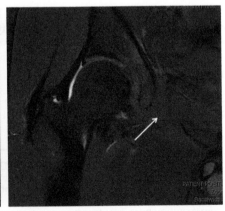

Fig. 1. 17-year-old lacrosse player with groin pain, diagnosed with superior acetabular labral tear. Tear pattern and clinical characteristics were not typical for symptomatic labral pathology, so repeat MRI with intravenous (IV) contrast was obtained 1 month later demonstrating Ewing sarcoma (*white arrow*).

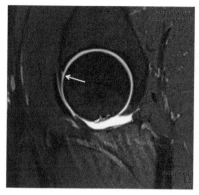 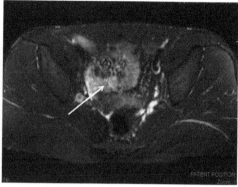

Fig. 2. 18-year-old soccer player with groin pain, diagnosed with an anterior labral tear on MRI (*arrow*). Also complained of lower abdominal pain and mild constitutional symptoms. Expanded MRI of the pelvis with intravenous contrast demonstrated signal enhancement and widespread bowel inflammation consistent with Crohn disease.

acetabular labral tears, chondral injuries, or even meniscal–chondral injuries of the knee.

LOCATION

The location of an athlete's hip pain should always be ascertained and may reveal important clues that reflect the etiology of the primary pain generator. A layer concept has been proposed to help clinicians understand the link between intra- and extra-articular pain generators, pain topography, and compensatory injury patterns.[2] Patients with an intra-articular pain source often describe the location of their pain in a C-shaped arc that courses from the anterior groin, over the lateral hip, to the buttock region. Although many potential injury patterns exist (and may coexist), anterior hip or groin pain should arouse suspicion of anterosuperior (ASIS) or anteroinferior (AIIS) iliac spine apophysitis, iliopsoas or adductor tenosynovitis, symptomatic femoroacetabular impingement (FAI) with anterosuperior chondro–labral injury, or athletic pubalgia.

Lateral hip pain should elicit concern for pathology within the abductor complex (gluteus medius and minimus, common in cross-country runners), trochanteric bursal irritation, or friction from iliotibial band (ITB) contracture. Adolescents with acetabular dysplasia frequently present with lateral hip pain caused by fatigue overload of the abductor complex secondary to poor lateral acetabular containment and stability. Although lateral hip pain has traditionally been associated with extra-articular pain generators, emerging knowledge suggests that intra-articular pathology may contribute to lateral hip pain much more commonly than previously believed.[3] Isolated posterior buttock pain may suggest lumbosacral pathology or deep gluteal pain syndrome with associated entrapment neuritis of the sciatic nerve, piriformis, and short external rotator contracture.

CHARACTER/QUALITY

The character and quality of pain may also help designate an appropriate diagnosis. Pain may be sharp and mechanical or dull and aching. Coxa saltans (ie, snapping hip syndrome) may be associated with iliopsoas contracture and tenosynovitis (anterior) or ITB contracture and abrasion (lateral). Patients with symptomatic ITB snapping often complain that their hip is dislocating and usually can reproduce their symptoms. Iliopsoas snapping is common in the setting of atraumatic hip instability because of anterior acetabular deficiency and increased secondary demand on the anterior hip capsule and anterior soft tissue stabilizers.[4] Catching or mechanical locking may result from unstable labral–chondral injury or intra-articular loose bodies. Pain that is of an aching quality may reflect synovitis, myofascial irritation, or stress reaction.

TEMPORAL FACTORS

The duration and factors associated with the production of pain are key elements of a thorough history. Most soft tissue sprains or minor myofascial injuries generally resolve over a 4- to 6-week course and should demonstrate consistent step-wise improvement. Injuries that persist beyond this period should motivate additional workup to evaluate for a more significant injury. Most hip pain is predominantly static or dynamic.[2] Dynamic pain is often reproduced with athletic training or functional sport-specific activities such as cutting, pivoting, impact landing, or explosive ballistic movements. Symptomatic FAI with labral–chondral injury, hip instability, or apophysitis characteristically produce a dynamic type of hip pain. Static pain often occurs in the absence of high-energy motion and may result from compromise of the neuroproprioceptive feedback arc or poor muscular coordination and cocontraction. Static pain may be associated with underlying systemic pain sources (eg, autoimmune, rheumatologic, connective tissue, or dysfunction).

PHYSICAL EXAMINATION

Physical examination of the young athlete with hip pain is essential to further support or refute the suspected diagnosis and gain a greater understanding of the anatomic contributors to hip dysfunction. A meticulous approach to examining the hip has been thoroughly described and proceeds in a layered approach.[5] A complete examination includes evaluation of gait and physical tests in the standing, seated, supine, decubitous (lateral), and prone. Specialized tests are utilized to clarify whether the pain source is intra- or extra-articular.

GAIT/STANDING

Antalgic gait patterns may include a hip-extension avoidance gait with decreased stride length. Limiting push-off and terminal extension is a protective mechanism to minimize pain from anterior capsular contracture and stretch on the irritable anterior soft tissues.[6] Abductor compromise may manifest as a Trendelenburg gait pattern, although this is less common in adolescents groups. Exceptions would include athletes suffering from chronic ITB contracture or snapping and abductor inhibition. Instructing the patient to attempt a single leg lunge may reveal subtle dynamic abductor imbalance manifesting as pelvic drop or lateral trunk flexion upon execution. In the standing position, patients with ITB contracture and snapping can usually reproduce their symptoms, producing a visually impressive snap as the contracted posterior third of the ITB subluxes back and forth across the greater trochanter.

SEATED/SUPINE

A seated examination forces the pelvis into a stable position and can be used to evaluate hip range of motion (ROM). Patients with deep gluteal pain syndromes often sit with an avoidance posture that limits direct pressure on the deep gluteal structures. Supine examination focuses on observation of skin and soft tissues for ecchymosis, abrasions, swelling, or gross deformity. High-energy bony or soft tissue avulsion injuries may incur significant disruption of surrounding vascular structures and produce bruising, hematoma, and swelling. Palpation of the iliac crest, ASIS, AIIS, ischium, pubis, and greater trochanteric physes may reveal point tenderness suspicious for avulsion injury. ROM testing should be repeated in the supine position and conducted with the contralateral hemipelvis stabilized. Comparative measurements should be taken and discrepancies noted. Leg lengths should be grossly assessed by comparing the height of the medial malleoli with the pelvis in the relaxed and balanced positions.

SPECIAL TESTS

Special examination tests can be used to differentiate between a variety of intra- or extra-articular pain generators.[7] A log-roll test is useful to detect capsulitis and can also reveal capsular contracture with FAI or severe synovitis. In a supine position, the affected hip is rolled back and forth, with the leg in a neutral position. Pain or limited motion constitutes a positive test. A similar dial test can be performed in the supine position to diagnose capsular laxity in patients with hip instability. An external rotation force is applied to the effected leg and released. Capsular tone is assessed visually as the leg rebounds into internal rotation (IR). Comparative testing is conducted on the contralateral limb, and if rebound IR is limited on the affected leg and is asymmetrical compared with the unaffected hip, the test is considered positive. Anterior impingement testing is generally performed to assess for anterosuperior labral–chondral injury and FAI. The affected hip is brought into flexion past 90° with variable degrees of IR and adduction (FADIR). A test is considered positive when pain is elicited and ROM compromised. The scour test is a dynamic test that places the hip into a similar provocative position with compression and sequential IR and external rotation (ER), producing pain in the presence of intra-articular pathology. FAI may effect the hip anteriorly with FADIR maneuvers or the lateral hip with a more lateral pattern of pathomorphology. Passive abduction with IR or ER would elicit pain and correspond with activity-related symptoms (horseback riding, martial arts, dance). Effectively, the zone of impingement can be dialed in based on the position of anatomic conflict or physical abutment during ROM testing. Pain primarily with straight and deep passive hip flexion may suggest an extra-articular source of impingement between the AIIS and femoral neck, and is common in dancers and martial artists. Manual muscle strength testing should be performed in the supine position with the knee both flexed and extended to isolated strength deficits of the hip flexor complex (tensor fascia lata [TFL] plus iliopsoas (IP) and rectus femoris) versus individual hip flexors.

Pain may also be generated with flexion, abduction, and ER (FABER). Posterior pain with FABER testing is usually associated with sacroilitis, while anterior hip pain is commonly attributed to iliofemoral ligament or iliopsoas contracture and tenosynovitis. A positive FABER test is associated with side-to-side asymmetry in ROM and pain. While performing FABER testing, a dynamic examination can be performed to assess for IP snapping. The hip is slowly brought from a position of slight flexion, abduction, and ER to extension and IR. A reproducible grinding, clicking, or clunking can be palpated and usually heard. This is typically painful for the patient. Pain with resisted abdominal activation and/or hip adduction suggests athletic pubalgia with injury to the rectus abdomens or tendinous origin of the adductor complex. In the supine position, abdominal lower quadrant palpation superior to the inguinal ligament should also be performed to determine if there may be abdominal visceral pathology contributing to pain.

DECUBITOUS/PRONE

With the patient lying on his or her side in a decubitous position, the abductor and deep gluteal complex can be palpated for points of tenderness indicating trochanteric bursal irritation, gluteus medius/minimus pathology, or piriformis/short external rotator irritation. The sacroiliac joint and lumbosacral spine can also be inspected in the lateral position. Ober test is performed by allowing the affected hip (top hip) to passively extend and assessing for contracture or inability to passively adduct. Manual muscle strength testing should be performed with the knee alternatively extended and flexed to isolate abductor complex strength (knee straight for glut max/TFL plus gluteus medius/minimus) versus isolated gluteus medius/minimus (knee flexed). Prone examination can be conducted to gain further clinical information on the integrity of the common hamstring (biceps femoris, semimembranosis, and semitendinosis), gluteal complex, and the ischial tuberosity.

IMAGING
Radiographs

Appropriate imaging of the injured adolescent hip and pelvis begins with a dedicated plain radiographic series.[8] A well centered anteroposterior (AP) pelvis (coccyx centered 1 cm above pubis without rotation) and cross-table or frog leg lateral view are essential for a basic radiographic interpretation of bony structures about the hip. Physeal injuries to the ASIS, iliac crest, ischial tuberosity, pubis, and greater and lesser trochanters can be detected on these views. SI joint narrowing or sclerosis (ankylosing spondylitis), and bony abnormalities of the iliac wings (bony lesions or traumatic injuries) are also apparent with this series. An AP pelvic radiograph provides a crude representation of acetabular version and proximal femoral geometry. Morphologic features characteristic of FAI (ie, Cam-type FAI: aspherical femoral head-neck junction, pistol-grip deformity, or decreased femoral head–neck offset; pincer-type FAI: cross-over sign, acetabular retroversion, ischial spine sign) are grossly depicted on AP and lateral views.[9] Acetabular volume, which is a proxy for femoral head containment or acetabular dysplasia, is represented by measuring a lateral center edge angle (LCEA). A false profile view is better suited to demonstrate ASIS or AIIS avulsion injuries and judge the degree of anterior acetabular coverage (anterior center-edge angle, ACEA). An extended femoral neck or Dunn view can be obtained with the hip flexed 45° or 90° and slightly abducted, to give a more accurate representation of Cam-type FAI variants with their characteristic femoral neck prominence (alpha angle >55°).

Ultrasound

Musculoskeletal ultrasound (MSUS) has emerged as a useful diagnostic tool with the ability to provide real-time dynamic imaging and feedback during provocative testing.[8] Advantages include convenient in-clinic use with the ability to perform diagnostic evaluation of both intra- and extra-articular structures with high definition. Disadvantages of MSUS include user dependence and a significant learning curve. Dynamic impingement and instability testing can be performed in real time with concomitant visualization of key periarticular soft tissues such as ITB and IP (Video 1). High-fidelity units can detect chondral, labral, and synovial abnormalities with high sensitivity and accuracy, and may eventually supplant the need for magnetic resonance imaging (MRI). MSUS also facilitates procedural interventions such as diagnostic and therapeutic intra- and extra-articular hip injections. Ultrasound-guided diagnostic injections are an extremely useful adjunct to clinical examination and can help identify the primary pain generator for a specific clinical scenario. Once an accurate diagnosis is established, an appropriate treatment strategy can be implemented.

Magnetic Resonance Imaging

Magnetic resonance imaging (MRI) and magnetic resonance arthrography (MRA) offer detailed information regarding the integrity of intra- and extra-articular soft tissue structures about the hip.[9] Traditional 1.5 T (1.5 T) and newer 3 T magnets produce high quality images and remain the gold standard for diagnosing acetabular labral and chondral pathology. Extra-articular injuries to the periarticular soft tissue envelope, stress reactions of the pelvis or hip, and intra-articular pathologies are all demonstrated with high diagnostic yield. The addition of intra-articular contrast, such as gadolinium, may further enhance the diagnostic accuracy of an MRI scan.[10] Several studies have demonstrated higher sensitivity and specificity and potential advantages of MRA over MRI for detection of intra-articular pathologies. However, with advances in imaging techniques and technology (3 T scanners), non-contrast magnetic resonance units are approaching equivalence for detecting intra-articular hip pathology.[11]

Computed Tomography

Computed tomography (CT) scans are most useful for characterization of bony avulsions or morphologic alterations in acetabular or proximal femoral anatomy. In the presence of FAI, CT scans can provide further definition of bony morphology and serve as a useful adjunct to other radiographic studies for preoperative tempting and planning (**Fig. 3**). Acetabular dysplasia may involve only a portion of the acetabulum or may be more global in its involvement. CT characterization is helpful to determine the severity of the dysplasia and for planning corrective osteotomies. Slices can be made through the distal femur to calculate proximal femoral version and should be considered, along with 3-dimensional reconstructions, to gain a complete understanding of the biomechanical influences on the weight-bearing articular surface of the hip joint.[12]

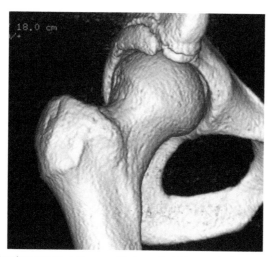

Fig. 3. Complex impingement pattern with type II AIIS morphology and mixed FAI with large structural acetabular rim fracture.

APOPHYSEAL INJURIES

Apophyseal or physeal injuries usually occur as the result of a sudden forceful contraction of the myotendinous complex that originates from its bony origin in that respective location. They are encountered frequently during sports such as soccer, gymnastics, or sprinting, which require rapid acceleration and deceleration. Repetitive stress to the epiphyseal plate may also produce a traction apophysitis that may present in a more insidious fashion. Various traumatic avulsion injuries are encountered, most commonly ischial avulsion fractures (54%), followed by AIIS (22%), and ASIS (19%) avulsions (**Fig. 4**).[13] Avulsion injuries may also occur with less frequency at the greater or lesser trochanters, iliac crest, or pubis (**Fig. 5**).

Young athletes who sustain an avulsion fracture often recall a single isolated noncontact event with acute onset of pain and functional weakness. There is often associated swelling, ecchymosis, and pain at the site of injury. Passive stretch or activation of the respective muscle group reproduces pain. Radiographic evaluation is generally sufficient to confirm the diagnosis and determine if operative or nonoperative treatment is appropriate.

Treatment

Athletes who sustain avulsion fractures with more than 2 cm displacement are considered for surgical reduction and stabilization, whereas avulsions with minimal displacement are generally treated conservatively (**Fig. 6**). For minimally displaced avulsions, treatment involves rest, activity modification, cryotherapy, and protected weight bearing. There is some evidence to support limiting the use of nonsteroidal anti-inflammatory drugs (NSAIDs) in the setting of fracture to minimize the potential

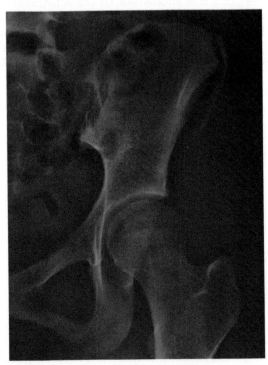

Fig. 4. Large iliac apophyseal avulsion in 14-year-old sprinter.

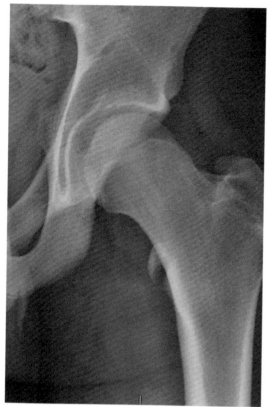

Fig. 5. Lesser trochanteric avulsion in 16-year-old soccer player with concomitant FAI morphology.

inhibitory effect of NSAIDs on primary bone healing.[14] Physical therapy can be initiated early to minimize disuse atrophy and compensatory gait and motion strategies and optimize functional recovery. Readiness to return to sports is predicated on restoration of motion, pain resolution, and successful completion of formal agility and sport-specific testing. Even when nonoperative treatment is indicated, sequelae of an overly exuberant biologic healing response may develop. Heterotopic bone formation (HO) can sometimes cause a compressive mass effect on surrounding neuromuscular or myotendinous structures when large enough. When HO occurs at the ischial tuberosity, late sciatic nerve entrapment and hamstring syndrome may develop and ultimately require surgical intervention (**Fig. 7**).[15] If HO forms at the site of a rectus femoris avulsion at the AIIS, an extra-articular pattern of impingement may develop between the femoral neck and malunited or deformed AIIS. In contrast, failure of primary bony union may also result in persistent pain and/or functional impairment, and require late surgical intervention to achieve definitive healing.

ACETABULAR LABRAL TEARS

Tears of the acetabular labrum have emerged as a significant source of intra-articular pain in the adolescent athlete over the last few decades. Improved imaging modalities, coupled with a growing clinical awareness have led to a rapid increase in diagnostic frequency.[16] The labrum is a horseshoe-shaped ring of fibrocartilage that surrounds

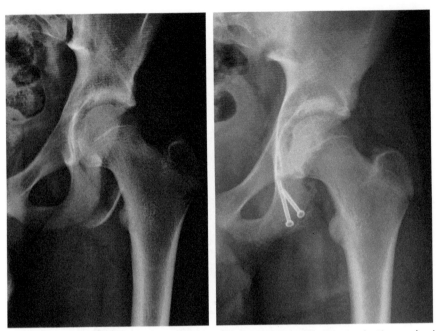

Fig. 6. Left ischial avulsion in a 14-year-old wrestler treated with open reduction and primary screw fixation.

the acetabulum, expanding the surface area of the joint and providing a suction seal, limiting cartilage consolidation and fluid egress. A watershed zone has been identified in the anterosuperior portion of the labrum, rendering this region vulnerable to injury. Labral tears exist as a spectrum, from focal labral bruising without frank

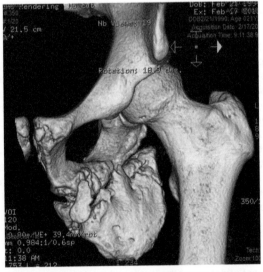

Fig. 7. Large focus of heterotopic bone formation with compressive mass effect, sequelae of an untreated hamstring avulsion. Treated with excision and proximal hamstring reconstruction.

labral–chondral separation, to more extensive injuries that involve the transitional labral–chondral interface, and even full separation of the labrum from its acetabular foundation.[17] Associated chondral pathology is almost always found in conjunction with labral tears. High-energy injuries with associated subluxation or dislocation events can produce acute traumatic tears, but these injury mechanisms are rare. More commonly, labral tears develop with insidious onset, as the result of repetitive loading and motion patterns, germane to a particular sport. Sports requiring high-energy mechanical stresses and rapid rotational movements may eventually lead to failure at the labral–chondral junction and pain. Labral tears are usually associated with underlying abnormal bony architecture, such as FAI or acetabular dysplasia, or more complex rotational deformities of the proximal femur or acetabulum.[18] An athlete with a symptomatic labral tear often complains of groin pain with strenuous or characteristic dynamic activities. There may be a pinching quality with deep hip flexion or rotation, and occasionally mechanical symptoms such as catching and locking may develop. As previously described, reliable physical examination findings include positive anterior impingement tests (FADIR or scour) and FABER maneuvers. MRI or MRA can be particularly helpful in confirming the diagnosis and may provide further information regarding concomitant chondral, bony, or periarticular soft tissue injury (**Fig. 8**).[17]

Treatment

Treatment is initiated by verifying that the labral tear visualized on MRI is truly symptomatic. Asymptomatic labral tears are very common in adult populations and are sometimes a red herring in younger athletic populations as well.[19] Ultrasound-guided intra-articular diagnostic injections can help differentiate intra- versus extra-articular pain.[8] To optimize nonoperative management, strenuous physical activity is curtailed, and a dedicated period of rest is usually initiated, along with a course of physical therapy. NSAIDs are often used to relieve the burden of pain associated with synovitis and compensatory periarticular muscle irritation. If an initial attempt (>3 months) at nonoperative treatment fails, referral to an arthroscopic hip surgeon

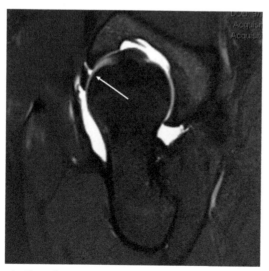

Fig. 8. MRA demonstrating a large anterosuperior labral tear (*arrow*) with transitional zone separation.

is reasonable, since continued pain and dysfunction can eventually lead to a host of compensatory injuries.[20] Technical innovations have enabled arthroscopic hip surgeons to treat labral and chondral pathology in creative new ways, with repair or refixation generally preferred over debridement whenever possible.[21] The number of arthroscopists performing hip arthroscopy and the number of annual hip arthroscopies performed per year have grown considerably in the last 10 years.[22] Favorable outcomes have been reported in adolescent populations in a number of observational cohort studies. When irreparable labral tears are encountered in young athletes, the labral sealing mechanism can be re-established using graft tissue (autograft or allograft; ITB, hamstring, tibialis anterior or posterior, ligamentum teres) to reconstruct the acetabular labrum.[23]

FEMOROACETABULAR IMPINGEMENT

FAI reflects a dynamic mechanical conflict between the quasi-hemispheric acetabulum and femoral neck (**Fig. 9**). FAI is predominantly conceptualized in 3 forms: Cam-type impingement (aspherical femoral head-neck junction), pincer-type (focal or global ace tabular retroversion or rim prominence), or a mixed-type (combined pathomorphology).[24] Most FAI is mixed-type and has been increasingly recognized as a potential contributor to progressive labral and chondral injury in the adolescent athlete. The theoretic link between FAI and idiopathic osteoarthritis in younger populations has been speculated for decades, but strong evidence has begun to emerge that supports this pathomechanical process.[25] Extra-articular forms of FAI are believed to exist as well and have received considerable attention in recent literature (iliopsoas, ischiofemoral, AIIS/subspine, trochanteric–pelvic impingement) (**Fig. 10**).[26]

Anatomic abutment or collision between the aspherical femoral neck and prominent acetabular rim is thought to cause labral and chondral injury, reduced functional ROM, and a dynamic source of pain for the athlete. Once recognized solely in young adult populations, FAI is now known to affect younger athletes also. Consequently, there is growing concern over the physical demands of high-level youth sports and the potential influence of these stresses on developing proximal femoral physes. Longitudinal studies have demonstrated a potential relationship between certain sports, such as youth hockey, and the development of FAI morphology over the course of years of training.[27] Moreover, cross-sectional studies have revealed a high rate of asymptomatic FAI among athletic populations.[28]

Young athletes with symptomatic FAI may present with a spectrum of complaints. In the earlier phase of onset, the athlete will sometimes only complain of pain during

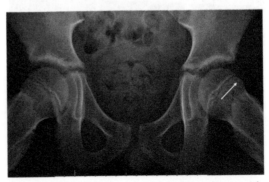

Fig. 9. Bilateral symptomatic FAI in a 9-year-old hockey player with plain radiographs revealing Cam-type morphology (*arrow*).

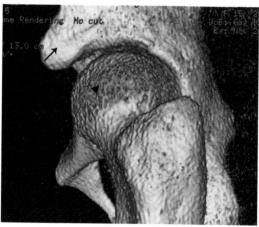

Fig. 10. Extra-articular subspine impingement caused by remote AIIS avulsion and subsequent healing. Note down-sloping AIIS (*arrow*) and linear damage of the femoral head (*arrowhead*) due to pathologic contact between the bony structures.

strenuous activity, but not at rest. Pain is usually concentrated around the groin area with frequent referral to the medial thigh or scrotum. In patients with later phase or more chronic presentations, there may be pain at rest, with prolonged sitting, or while standing. More lateral or posterior Cam lesions usually produce lateral or posterior pain with reduced abduction and external rotation. Physical examination findings are generally similar to those encountered with labral tears, with positive provocative anterior impingement tests, capsulitis, and reduced ROM. Imaging reveals reduced femoral head–neck offset or pistol-grip deformity, overcoverage of the acetabulum, and disruption of the labral–chondral junction on MRI.

Treatment

With the understanding that many athletes train and compete symptom free with clinically silent FAI, there is a role for initial conservative management of FAI. This includes restriction from sport, physical therapy with avoidance of engaging the hip in a position of functional impingement, NSAIDs, and modalities.[20] Consideration may be given to administering an intra-articular corticosteroid injection to alleviate pain and facilitate completion of a season, but this should be viewed as a bridging procedure that is unlikely to produce long-term benefit.[29] Surgical management of adolescent athletes with FAI is aimed at restoring normal bony morphology while simultaneously addressing labral–chondral injuries (**Fig. 11**). Both arthroscopic and open techniques have been applied with favorable results reported, and a low complication rate.[30,31] Several studies have compared clinical outcomes and accuracy of morphologic correction between open and arthroscopic techniques, and have been shown to be equivalent.[32] However, open techniques are often criticized for their increased soft tissue morbidity and potential for complications such as nonunion of their obligate trochanteric osteotomy. A high rate of return to sport has also been reported for adolescent athlete populations.

ATHLETIC PUBALGIA

Athletic pubalgia is a more recent term adopted in favor of the more traditional diagnosis sports hernia. Often used to describe a wide constellation of pathoanatomical

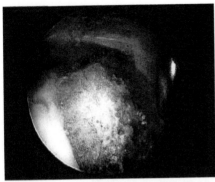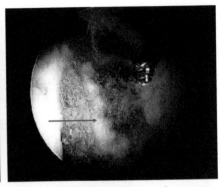

Fig. 11. Arthroscopic view of a Cam-lesion in a skeletally immature athlete with symptomatic FAI. Note the immature proximal femoral physis exposed after femoral head–neck osteochondroplasty (*red arrow*).

features, athletic pubalgia is characterized by central core dysfunction, and associated bony and/or soft tissue manifestations. The watershed zone at the central portion of the pelvis contains the myotendinous insertions of the rectus abdominus, the adductor complex (adductor longus, brevis, and pectineus), and the junction of the pubis (pubic symphysis). Both chronic overuse patterns of injury and acute traumatic mechanisms have been described (**Fig. 12**). This anatomic region is a central link in the kinetic chain, and sometimes referred to as the pelvic joint.[33] Injuries to the central core are often the result of repetitive overuse activities that involve engagement of the core muscles during dynamic athletic movements. Patients often describe groin pain or central pelvic pain of insidious onset that is reproduced with activation of the core muscles during activities such as sit-ups, coughing, or sneezing. Clinically, patients have pain on palpation at the pubic symphysis or bony insertions of the central core muscles. This pain is usually exacerbated by having the patient perform a resisted sit-up or adduction of the affected leg. Plain radiographs and CT are useful for characterizing bony avulsions, and MSUS can demonstrate dynamic pelvic floor weakness. MRI remains the imaging modality of choice for its wide view of the central pelvic structures and ability to detect bony edema and soft tissue pathologies.[34]

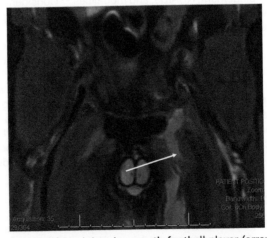

Fig. 12. Adductor sleeve avulsion injury in a youth football player (*arrow*).

Treatment

Like most other hip and pelvic injuries in adolescent athletes, an initial attempt at conservative management strategy is usually employed with relative rest, NSAIDs, and targeted physiotherapy. Ultrasound-guided injections of corticosteroid or biologic agents (platelet-rich plasma, or stem cell therapy) may be useful to help the athlete recover function without surgical intervention. Recent biomechanical studies have drawn a causative relationship between FAI morphology and increased stress on the central core. Clinical studies have also shown a high incidence of concomitant FAI and athletic pubalgia, and have recommended that whenever these pathologies coexist and require surgical treatment, both pathologies should be addressed simultaneously.[35] Surgery to address athletic pubalgia can reflect a number of isolated or combined repair techniques. Exploration and reinforcement of the pelvic floor or posterior inguinal wall can be performed laparoscopically or open, with or without mesh reinforcement. Some surgeons advocate a more comprehensive approach with concomitant repair or debridement of the pubic symphysis, adductor sleeve complex, rectus abdominus insertion, and surrounding neurolysis and denervation of the local sensory nerves. Favorable outcomes have been reported after open or laparoscopic groin repair as well as combined arthroscopic FAI decompression with labral repair and sports hernia repair.

COXA SALTANS (SNAPPING HIP) AND INSTABILITY

Snapping hip conditions can either be primary and isolated, without coexisting pathoanatomy, or be causally related to underlying structural instability of the hip joint. Traditionally, coxa saltans (snapping hip) was described as being intra-articular (intra-articular loose bodies, unstable labral–chondral injuries), external (ITB or gluteus maximus contracture and abrasion and snapping over the greater trochanter), or internal (Iliopsoas friction and snapping over the femoral head, iliopectineal eminence, or AIIS).[36] Recent studies have led to an improved understanding of the relationship between insufficient bony stability (borderline dysplasia), soft tissue laxity, and their effect on surrounding periarticular soft tissue structures.[37] When there is deficient containment of the femoral head by the acetabulum, there is a compensatory increase in the demand on the hip joint capsule and surrounding dynamic stabilizers (iliopsoas and abductor complex). Excessive proximal femoral anteversion can similarly increase the anterior shear vector on the joint and lead to anterior capsular attenuation. Dysfunctional gait and movement patterns can result, and, consequently, the ITB or IP may become contracted and produce painful mechanical snapping during stereotyped motions. Athletes who rely on a supraphysiologic ROM to train or compete are predisposed to snapping hip conditions. For example, a high rate of asymptomatic ITB and IP snapping is reported in dancers.[38]

In cases of clinically significant snapping, requesting that an athlete reproduce his or her symptoms often provides clues to the location of mechanical abrasion. If the ITB or gluteus maximus is snapping, the athlete will often flare his or her affected hip to the side, volitionally subluxing the posterior one-third of the ITB over the greater trochanter. Patients will often describe their hip as dislocating, although this is not the case. This reproducible subluxation is visually striking. In contrast, snapping that originates from the IP is often clearly audible, producing a low thunk or grinding as the athlete brings his or her hip from deep flexion, into external rotation and extension with internal rotation. It is important to inquire whether there is pain associated with this motion, because many young female athletes experience asymptomatic snapping. Intra-articular snapping is usually less predictable and is experienced as

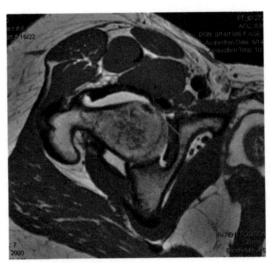

Fig. 13. Iliopsoas contracture with painful snapping and abrasion on femoral head articular cartilage demonstrated on MRI (*red arrow*).

a sudden sharp groin pain that causes the affected leg to buckle or give out. Plain radiographs and CT sans are useful to detect bony insufficiencies that may perpetuate atraumatic instability, and MRI can demonstrate capsular attenuation, labral–chondral pathology, or trochanteric bursal irritation. Dynamic ultrasound is particularly useful to document abnormal IP or ITB tracking and associated friction.[8,38]

Initial treatment of coxa saltans consists of rest from training and competition, NSAIDs, and physiotherapy to correct dysfunctional gait and movement patterns. When conservative modalities fail to provide long-term therapeutic benefit, surgery is indicated. Both open and arthroscopic techniques are described to fractionally lengthen the ITB (or gluteus maximus) and IP.[36] During endoscopic treatment of ITB snapping, coexistent trochanteric bursal scarring and adhesions can be removed through subcentimeter incisions. A high rate of good/excellent outcomes has been reported. The IP can be released at the level of the lesser trochanter, or through a trans-capsular window. Concomitant intra-articular pathology is addressed simultaneously. Contracture of the IP can cause injury to the labrum in some cases through a mechanism referred to as iliopsoas impingement (**Fig. 13**).[39] In the presence of capsular attenuation, arthroscopic capsular plication may be employed to achieve capsular volume reduction, effectively limiting extremes of motion and improving joint stability.[4]

SUPPLEMENTARY DATA

Supplementary data related to this article can be found online at http://dx.doi.org/10.1016/j.pcl.2014.08.004.

REFERENCES

1. Stanley E, Thigpen C. Throwing injuries in the adolescent athletes. Int J Sports Phys Ther 2013;8(5):630–40.
2. Draovitch P, Edelstein J, Kelly BT. The layer concept: utilization in determining pain generators, pathology, and how structure determines treatment. Curr Rev Musculoskelet Med 2012;5(1):1–8.

3. Domb BG, Botser I, Giordano BD. Outomes of endoscopic gluteus medius repair with 2-year follow-up. Am J Sports Med 2013;41(5):988–97.

4. Domb BG, Philippon MJ, Giordano BD. Arthroscopic capsulotomy, capsular repair, and capsular plication of the hip: relation to atraumatic instability. Arthroscopy 2013;29(1):162–73.

5. Martin HD, Kelly BT, Leunig M, et al. The pattern and technique in the clinical examination of the adult hip: the common physical examination tests of hip specialists. Arthroscopy 2010;26(2):161–72.

6. Bowman KF Jr, Fox J, Sekiya JK. A clinically relevant review of hip biomechanics. Arthroscopy 2010;26(8):1118–29.

7. Martin HD, Palmer IJ. History and physical examination of the hip: the basics. Curr Rev Musculoskelet Med 2013;6(3):219–25.

8. Jacobson JA, Bedi A, Sekiya JK, et al. Evaluation of the painful athletic hip. Imaging options and image-guided injections. AJR Am J Roentgenol 2012;199(3):516–24.

9. Nepple JJ, Prather H, Trousdale RT, et al. Diagnostic imaging of femoroacetabular impingement. J Am Acad Orthop Surg 2013;21(Suppl 1):S20–6.

10. Sutter R, Zubler V, Hoffman A, et al. Hip MRI: how useful is intraarticular contrast material for evaluating surgically proven lesions of the labrum and articular cartilage? AJR Am J Roentgenol 2014;202(1):160–9.

11. Robinson P. Conventional 3-T MRI and 1.5-T MR arthrography of femoroacetabular impingement. AJR Am J Roentgenol 2012;199(3):509–15.

12. Botser IB, Ozoude GC, Martin DE. Femoral anteversion in the hip: comparison of measurement by computed tomography, magnetic resonance imaging, and physical examination. Arthroscopy 2012;28(5):619–27.

13. Rossi F, Dragoni S. Acute aculsion fractures of the pelvis in adolescent competitive athletes: prevalence, location, and sports distribution of 203 cases collected. Skeletal Radiol 2001;30(3):127–31.

14. Geusens P, Emans PJ, de Jong JJ, et al. NSAIDs and fracture healing. Curr Opin Rheumatol 2013;25(4):524–31.

15. Bowman KF Jr, Cohen SB, Bradley JP. Operative management of partial-thickenss tears of the proximal hamstring muscle in athletes. Am J Sports Med 2013;41(6):1363–71.

16. Safran MR. The acetabular labrum: anatomic and functional characteristics and rationale for surgical intervention. J Am Acad Orthop Surg 2010;18(6):338–45.

17. Czerny C, Hofman S, Urban M, et al. MR arthrography of the adult acetabular capsular–labral complex: correlation with surgery and anatomy. AJR Am J Roentgenol 1999;173(2):345–9.

18. Wenger DE, Kendell KR, Miner MR, et al. Acetabular labral tears rarely occur in the absence of bony abnormalities. Clin Orthop Relat Res 2004;426:145–50.

19. Register B, Pennock AT, Ho CP, et al. Prevalence of abnormal hip findings in asymptomatic participants: a prospective blinded study. Am J Sports Med 2012;40(12):2720–4.

20. Wall PD, Fernandez M, Griffin DR, et al. Non-operative treatment for femoroacetabular impingement. A systematic review of the literature. PM R 2013;5(5):218–26.

21. Larson CM, Giveans MR, Stone RM. Arthroscopic debridement versus refixation of the acetabular labrum associated with femoroacetabular impingement: mean 3.5-year follow-up. Am J Sports Med 2012;40(5):1015–21.

22. Bozik KJ, Chan V, Valone FH, et al. Trends in hip arthroscopy utilization in the United States. J Arthroplasty 2013;28(8):140–3.

23. Ayeni OR, Alradwan H, de Sa D, et al. The hip labrum reconstruction: indications and outcomes—a systemic review. Knee Surg Sports Traumatol Arthrosc 2014; 22(4):737–43.
24. Byrd JW. Femoroacetabular impingement in athletes: part 1. Cause and assessment. Sports Health 2010;2(4):321–33.
25. Ganz R, Parvizi J, Beck M, et al. Femoroacetabular impingement: a cause for osteoarthritis of the hip. Clin Orthop Relat Res 2003;417:112–20.
26. Leunig M, Ganz R. The evolution and concepts of joint-preserving surgery of the hip. J Bone Joint Surg Br 2014;96B(1):5–18.
27. Philippon MJ, Ho CP, Briggs KK, et al. Prevalence of increased alpha angles as a measure of Cam-type femoroacetabular impingement in youth ice-hockey players. Am J Sports Med 2013;41(6):1357–62.
28. Nepple JJ, Brophy RH, Matava MJ, et al. Radiographic findings of femoroacetabular impingement in National Football League Combine athletes undergoing radiographs for previous hip or groin pain. Arthroscopy 2012;28(10):1396–403.
29. Krych AJ, Griffith TB, Hudgens JL, et al. Limited therapeutic benefits of intra-article cortisone injection for patients with femoro–acetabular impingement and labral tear. Knee Surg Sports Traumatol Arthrosc 2014;22(4):750–5.
30. Philippon MJ, Yen YM, Briggs KK, et al. Early outcomes after hip arthroscopy for femoroacetabular impingement in the athletic adolescent patient: a preliminary report. J Pediatr Ophthalmol 2008;28(7):705–10.
31. Naal FD, Miozzari HH, Wyss TF, et al. Surgical hip dislocation for the treatment of femoroacetabular impingement in high-level athletes. Am J Sports Med 2011; 39(3):544–50.
32. Matsuda DK, Carlisle JC, Arthurs SC, et al. Comparative systematic review of the open dislocation, mini-open, and arthroscopic surgeries for femoroacetabular impingement. Arthroscopy 2011;27(2):252–69.
33. Meyers WC, McKechnie A, Philippon MJ, et al. Experience with "sports hernia" spanning two decades. Ann Surg 2008;248(4):656–65.
34. Mullens FE, Zoga AC, Morrison WB, et al. Review of MRI technique and imaging findings in athletic pubalgia and the "sport hernia". Eur J Radiol 2012;81(12): 3780–92.
35. Larson CM, Pierce BR, Giveans MR. Treatment of athletes with symptomatic intra-articular hip pathology and athletic pubalgia/sports hernia: a case series. Arthroscopy 2011;27(6):768–75.
36. Ilizaliturri VM Jr, Camacho-Galindo J. Endoscopic treatment of snapping hips, iliotibial band, and iliopsoas tendon. Sports Med Arthrosc 2010;18(2):120–7.
37. Fabricant PD, Bedi A, De La Torre K, et al. Clinical outcomes after arthroscopic psoas lengthening: the effect of femoral version. Arthroscopy 2012;28(7):965–71.
38. Winston P, Awan R, Cassidy JD, et al. Clinical examination and ultrasound of self-reported snapping hip syndrome in elite ballet dancers. Am J Sports Med 2007; 35(1):118–26.
39. Domb BG, Shindle MK, McArthur B, et al. Iliopsoas impingement: a newly identified cause of labral pathology in the hip. HSS J 2011;7(2):145–50.

Assessment and Treatment of Knee Pain in the Child and Adolescent Athlete

Yi-Meng Yen, MD, PhD

KEYWORDS

- Patellofemoral • Injury • Ligament tear • Pediatrics

KEY POINTS

- A patient's description of knee pain is helpful in focusing the differential diagnosis.
- A good history and physical examination, followed by appropriate imaging is paramount for the diagnosis. Always check and examine the hip joint as well.
- A history of locking episodes could suggest meniscal injury or plica.
- A sensation of popping at the time of injury suggests a ligamentous injury. Giving way of the knee may represent ligamentous injury, patellar subluxation or dislocation, or even quadriceps inhibition or malfunction.

INTRODUCTION

Knee pain is one of the most common musculoskeletal complaints seen in the pediatric and adolescent population. The complaint is most prevalent in physical active patients, with up to 54% of athletes having some degree of knee pain per year.[1] The knee is a trocho-ginglymus joint allowing flexion and extension as well as slight internal and external rotation. The 2 joints within the knee consist of the patellofemoral articulation between the patella and femur and the tibiofemoral joint between the tibia and femur. A fairly extensive differential diagnosis exists for knee pain and can present a challenge to physicians. A detailed history, focused physical examination, and, when indicated, appropriate use of imaging modalities and laboratory tests can lead to accurate diagnosis and treatment.

Assessment

A patient's description of knee pain is helpful in focusing the differential diagnosis. As with any patient evaluation, a history of the pain must be elicited and should include the characteristics of the pain, onset (acute or insidious), location, duration, severity,

Disclosure: None.
Division of Sports Medicine, Boston Children's Hospital, Harvard Medical School, 300 Longwood Avenue, Boston, MA 02115, USA
E-mail address: Yi-Meng.Yen@childrens.harvard.edu

Pediatr Clin N Am 61 (2014) 1155–1173
http://dx.doi.org/10.1016/j.pcl.2014.08.003
0031-3955/14/$ – see front matter
pediatric.theclinics.com

quality, and radiation. Aggravating or alleviating factors should be identified, and if the knee pain was caused by acute injury, the ability to weight bear after the injury should be discerned. Mechanical symptoms, such as locking, popping, catching, or giving way of the knee, should be ascertained. A history of locking episodes could suggest meniscal injury or plica. A sensation of popping at the time of injury suggests a ligamentous injury. Giving way of the knee may represent ligamentous injury, patellar subluxation or dislocation, or even quadriceps inhibition or malfunction. A history of prior knee injury or surgery is important, as is a history of rheumatologic disease.

The presence of an effusion is important to note for knee pain. Rapid onset of effusion after an acute injury suggests a hemarthrosis and could represent fracture or cruciate ligament injury. A slow onset of effusion may represent meniscal injury or ligament sprain. An effusion in the absence of injury may indicate infection. If an acute injury occurred, the patient should be questioned about the specific mechanism of injury. It is important to determine if there was a direct blow, the direction of the blow, if the foot was planted at the time of injury, if the patient was accelerating or decelerating, a twisting component, or if landing from a jump. An anterior blow to the tibia with the knee in flexion can cause posterior cruciate ligament (PCL) injury. A valgus force produces a medial collateral ligament (MCL) injury whereas a varus force produces a lateral collateral ligament (LCL) injury. The anterior cruciate ligament (ACL) can be ruptured with a deceleration, hyperextension, and rotational injury. A rotational injury can also cause meniscal damage or patella subluxation. Any of these forces in children could produce fractures other than ligamentous injury due to the relative strength of the ligament compared with bone in this age group.

Physical Examination

The physician begins the examination of the knee by starting at the more proximal joint, the hip. Pain from the hip can be perceived as knee pain, likely due to the innervation of the anterior branch of the obturator nerve or articular branches of the femoral, common peroneal, or saphenous nerves.[2] It is, therefore, mandatory that a complete examination of the hip accompany an examination of the knee. The knee evaluation is conducted by comparing the asymptomatic knee to the painful one. The injured knee is inspected for erythema, bruising, swelling, and discoloration. The musculature around the knee should be symmetric on both sides, and, in particular, the vastus medialis obilquus should be noted for any signs of atrophy.

The knee is then palpated, and areas of tenderness should be noted, particularly at the tibial tubercle, patella, joint line, and femoral condyle in flexion. The patella should be checked to see if it is ballotable, indicating effusion of the joint, and any warmth of the knee noted. Range of motion should be examined by flexing and extending the knee as far as possible. During the range-of-motion examination, patellofemoral tracking should be noted and the presence of crepitus detected. The Q-angle can be determined by drawing a line from the anterior superior iliac crest through the center of the patella and a second line from the center of the patella to the tibial tuberosity. A Q-angle greater than 15° may be a predisposing factor for patella maltracking. A J-sign is noted, which is the movement of the patella laterally on terminal extension of the knee. Patella mobility can be assessed both laterally and medially, in which one quadrant of motion is considered normal, and a patellar apprehension test can be performed. With a laterally directed force on the medial aspect of the patella, the physician attempts to subluxate the patella from 0° to 90°. If this reproduces a patient's pain or feeling of giving way, this test is positive.[3]

Assessment of the cruciate ligaments begins with the knee flexed at 90° (**Table 1**). Normally, the medial tibial plateau extends 1 cm anteriorly beyond the femoral condyle

Table 1
Physical examination maneuvers

Test	Description	
ACL tests		
Anterior drawer test	Patient is supine, hip flexed to 45° and knee flexed to 90°. Examiner sits on patient's foot with hands behind proximal tibia and thumbs on tibial plateau. Anterior force is applied, increased tibial translation compared with other sides is indicative of tear.	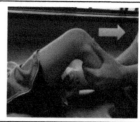
Lachman test	Patient is supine, knee at 15° of flexion. Femur is stabilized with one hand while other hand stabilizes tibia. Femur is pushed posterior and tibia is pulled anteriorly. Increased translation and soft endpoint are indicative of a positive test.	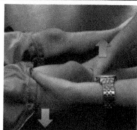
PCL tests		
Posterior drawer	Patient is supine, hip flexed to 45° and knee flexed to 90°. Examiner sits on patient's foot with hands behind proximal tibia and thumbs on tibial plateau. Posterior force is applied, increased tibial translation compared with other sides is indicative of tear.	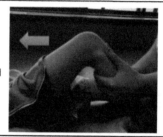
MCL and LCL tests		
Valgus stress test	Patient supine, knee flexed to 30°, hands on both sides of tibia, fingers used to stabilize femur. Application of valgus stress, if increased translation, indicative of MCL injury.	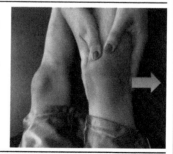

(continued on next page)

Table 1
(continued)

Test	Description	
Varus stress test	Patient supine, knee flexed to 30°, hands on both sides of tibia, fingers used to stabilize femur. Application of valgus stress, if increased translation, indicative of LCL injury.	
Meniscal tests		
McMurray test	Patient is supine, the knee is fully flexed. Foot is held by the heel. The leg is rotated on the thigh with the knee in full flexion by internally and externally rotating. Altering the degree of flexion allows the whole segment of meniscus to be examined. If a click occurs, the test is considered positive.	

when the knee is flexed to 90°.[4] Posterior displacement of the tibia indicates a torn PCL. Next, the examiner sits on the foot and positions a hand behind the proximal tibia with the thumbs on the tibial plateau. A posterior directed force assesses for the posterior displacement of the tibia; increased posterior displacement compared with the contralateral side is indicative of a partial or complete tear of the PCL. An anterior drawer test can also performed, which can compare anterior displacement of the tibia with the uninjured side. Increased anterior displacement suggests ACL disruption. Chronic injuries tend to be more sensitive to the anterior drawer test than acute injuries.[5–7] In general, the Lachman and pivot shift tests are both more sensitive and specific to ACL injuries[5–10] and are the preferred tests to the anterior drawer. The Lachman test is performed with a patient in the supine position and the knee flexed to 30°. The examiner stabilizes the distal femur with one hand and the proximal tibia with the other. The tibia is then attempted to be subluxated anteriorly; lack of a clear endpoint to translation or increased translation compared with the uninjured side is indicative of a positive test.

The collateral ligaments are tested with a patient's leg in slight adduction. The examiner places one hand on the lateral aspect of the knee joint and the other hand on the medial aspect of the proximal tibia. Valgus stress is applied at the knee at both full extension and at 30°. Laxity of the tibia or absence of an endpoint on examination indicates disruption of the MCL at 30°; at full extension, it indicates disruption of the MCL and one of the cruciate ligaments.[11] Varus stress testing is similar to valgus stress testing except the examiner's one hand is placed on the medial aspect of the knee joint and the other hand on the lateral aspect of the proximal fibula.

Patients with injury to the meniscus usually demonstrate tenderness at the medial or lateral joint line.[12,13] Flexion of the knee enhances the palpation of the anterior portion of both menisci. The McMurray test as originally described involves the patient supine with the knee fully flexed.[14] With the knee in flexion, the tibia is rotated internally to test for the posterior horn of the lateral meniscus and externally rotated to test for the medial meniscus. An appreciable snap is considered positive and indicative of a torn meniscus. By altering the position of flexion, the whole of the posterior segment of meniscus can be examined (see **Table 1**).

Protocols have been developed to try to reduce the number of radiographs used in the evaluation of extremity injuries. The two best-known guidelines are the Ottawa knee rules and the Pittsburgh rules.[15–18] In a prospective study, the Pittsburgh rules were more specific and sensitive than the Ottawa rules.[19] If using the Pittsburgh rules, the inability to bear weight, effusion, or ecchymosis is an indication to obtain antero-posterior, sunrise, and lateral radiographs of the knee (**Box 1**). In patients with chronic knee pain and recurrent effusions, a notch or tunnel view (posteroanterior view of the knee flexed to 40°–50°) should be obtained. Clinical judgment should always be used, however, for the determination if radiographs are necessary. If radiographs are inconclusive, advanced imaging, such as MRI, may be necessary.

The presence of warmth, nontraumatic effusion, or significant pain with slight range of motion may be consistent with septic arthritis or an acute inflammatory arthropathy. In these cases, the use of laboratory studies is indicated. A complete blood cell count, sedimentation rate, and C-reactive protein should be obtained. Additionally, in endemic regions, a Lyme disease titer should be sent. An arthrocentesis may be required to differentiate the diagnosis (**Table 2**). The presence of a hemarthrosis indicates a fracture or ligamentous injury. Clear fluid suggests a sprain or possible chronic injury, whereas purulent fluid indicates infection. The joint fluid should be sent to a laboratory for a cell count with differential, glucose, and protein measurements; bacterial culture and sensitivity; and, in certain instances, the testing for crystals.

OVERUSE INJURY
Osteochondrosis

Osgood-Schlatter

Osgood-Schlatter disease is a common cause of anterior knee pain in children and adolescents. It is caused by repetitive traction of the patellar tendon on the tibial

---

Box 1
Decision rules for knee radiographs

Ottawa knee rules

  Age greater than 55 years

  Isolated tenderness of the patella

  Tenderness at the head of the fibula

  Inability to flex knee to 90°

  Inability to bear weight immediately after injury AND in an emergency department for 4 steps

Pittsburgh knee rules

  Blunt trauma or fall as mechanism of injury AND

    Age less than 12 or greater than 50 years

    Inability to walk 4 full weight-bearing steps in the ED

Table 2
Synovial fluid findings

Classification	Condition	Color	Clarity	WBC/μL	Neutrophil (%)	Crystals	Culture
Normal	Clear	Yellow	Transparent	<200	<25	−	−
Noninflammatory	Osteoarthritis	Yellow	Transparent	<2000	<25	−	−
	Trauma	Pink or red	Translucent	<2000	<25	−	−
Inflammatory	Rheumatoid arthritis	Yellowish	Translucent or opaque	3000–50,000	50–75	−	−
	Gout	Yellow or white	Translucent or opaque	100–160,000	90	+	−
	Lupus	Yellow	Translucent	0–9000	<25	−	−
Infectious	Lyme[20–22]	Yellow	Opaque	10,000–100,000	>85	−	−
	Bacterial	Yellowish	Opaque	50,000–300,000	>90	−	+

Abbreviation: WBC, white blood cell.

tubercle ossification center. Symptomatic patients are typically between the ages of 8 and 14, and 30% of patients have bilateral knee involvement.[23,24] Symptoms are typically exacerbated with activities that involve jumping (basketball, volleyball, and running) or with direct contact of the tubercle (kneeling).[25] Radiographic evaluation of early Osgood-Schlatter demonstrates irregularity of the apophysis with separation from the tibial tubercle, whereas late disease shows fragmentation of the apophysis (**Fig. 1**).

The standard of treatment of Osgood-Schlatter is nonoperative and includes icing, limitation of activities, oral antiinflammatory medication, physical therapy, and knee bracing.[24,26–29] Generally, Osgood-Schlatter runs a self-limiting course with complete recovery expected with closure of the tibial growth plate. In rare recalcitrant cases, surgical excision of the ossicle can give good pain relief in skeletally mature patients.[30,31]

Sinding-Larsen-Johansson

Another common cause of anterior knee pain may be Sinding-Larsen-Johansson disease, which results from persistent traction at the inferior pole of the patella, leading to calcification and ossification at that junction.[32] Symptomatic patients are usually between the ages of 10 and 12 who complain of activity-related pain, particularly with jumping, running, and kneeling. The pain and swelling are localized to the inferior pole of the patella. Radiographic evaluation can show variable amount of calcification or ossification at the inferior pole of the patella (**Fig. 2**).

Treatment is similar to that of Osgood-Schlatter, with icing, limitation of activity, nonsteroidal antiinflammatory drugs, or knee sleeve as the standard of treatment. This condition is benign and self-limiting and almost always resolves without sequelae and surgery is rarely needed.

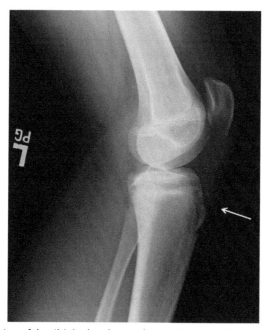

Fig. 1. Fragmentation of the tibial tubercle apophysis indicative of late stage Osgood-Shlatter disease. Arrow shows ossicle of bone at tibial tuberosity.

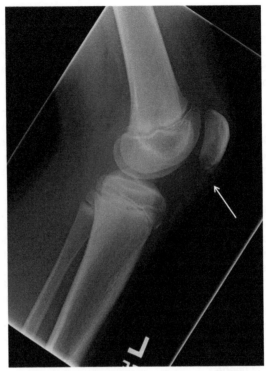

Fig. 2. Fragmentation of the inferior pole of the patella in Sinding-Larsen-Johansson. Arrow shows ossicle of bone at inferior pole of patella.

Synovial Plicae of the Knee

Synovial plicae may cause anterior knee pain in children and adolescents. Plica syndrome can present with anterior knee pain and clicking, catching, locking, or pseudo-locking of the knee. An acute injury to the plica may cause inflammation and exacerbate symptoms. It is believed that the symptoms are caused by the bowing of the plica across the femoral condyle on flexion of the knee.[33,34] During embryonic development, the knee is compartmentalized by suprapatellar, medial, and lateral synovial septae. With further development, depending on the degree of septal recession, persistence of the infrapatellar, suprapatellar, lateral, or medial plica can remain. The infrapatellar and suprapatellar plicae likely do not cause significant symptoms, and the lateral plica is exceedingly rare.[35,36]

The medial plica is the one that most frequently produces the symptoms of chronic anterior knee pain. Often there is a history of striking the anteromedial aspect of the knee followed by a chronic aching of the knee made worse with activity. Tenderness around the medial plica, which is commonly 1 fingerbreadth proximal and medial to the inferior pole of the patella, can suggest plica syndrome. Typically there is minimal effusion and the plica causes pain when palpated and rolled over the medial femoral condyle. Occasionally, there can be popping at approximately 30° to 40° of knee flexion.[37] Radiographs are negative, but MRI can demonstrate the presence of a plica. Routine use of MRI to detect a plica is not, however, recommended.

Treatment of synovial plica should be conservative. Modification of activity to reduce repetitive flexion and extension, physical therapy, and nonsteroidal antiinflammatory drugs should be used. Conservative management often leads to sufficient reduction in the synovitis and edema so that the plica resumes a more normal resiliency and no longer produces symptoms. Surgery should be reserved for those patients in whom other diagnoses have been ruled out and who have failed all modes of conservative management. Arthroscopic management of symptomatic plicae of the knee has been shown successful.[38,39]

Osteochondritis Dissecans

Osteochondritis dissecans (OCD) has been described as an acquired, potentially reversible, idiopathic lesion of subchondral bone resulting in the delamination and sequestration with or without corresponding articular cartilage involvement and instability.[40–43] The cause of OCD remains unknown, although multiple theories have been entertained. The juvenile form most commonly affects the lateral aspect of the medial femoral condyle, although lesions can occur on the lateral femoral condyle and the patellofemoral joint. Patients often report a vague, poorly localized knee pain, with recurrent effusion. If the articular cartilage becomes unstable and breaks off, the corresponding loose body can create mechanical symptoms of locking or catching of the knee.

Physical examination of the knee often reveals quadriceps atrophy and tenderness along the surface of the affected chondral area with deep palpation. A small joint effusion may be present. Radiographs can be diagnostic and should include the anteroposterior, lateral, Merchant, and notch or tunnel views. MRI is highly sensitive in detecting these lesions and can help determine if the OCD is radiographically stable or unstable (**Fig. 3**).

Treatment of small stable juvenile OCD lesions begins with 6 to 8 weeks of limited weight bearing or even immobilization, followed by unloader bracing and activity restriction.[44] Lesions that fail conservative treatment, large lesions, or unstable OCD

A   **B**

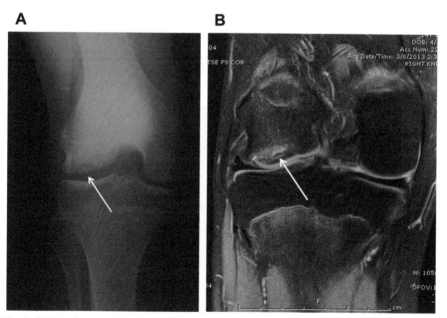

Fig. 3. (A) Notch view of the knee showing OCD lesion of the lateral femoral condyle. Arrow denotes OCD lesion. (B) T2-weighted MRI of the same OCD lesion; arrow denotes fluid undercutting lesion indicating an unstable OCD.

can be treated with operative intervention. Antegrade or retrograde drilling of the lesion, screw fixation, curettage and bone graft, microfracture, autologous chondrocyte implantation, osteochondral autograft, and allograft have all been used as treatment options with varying degrees of success.[45–52]

TRAUMATIC INJURY
Fracture

Sleeve fracture
Avulsion fractures of the inferior or superior pole of the patella are rare and constitute approximately 1% of all children's fractures.[53] The low incidence of fractures may be a result of less stress loads and pressure on the patella due to the flexible soft tissue and mobile nature of the patella. Additionally, the thick layer of cartilage may act as a cushion to a direct blow. A superior avulsion fracture involves the superior pole of the patella is a more uncommon fracture pattern.[54] An inferior avulsion injury involves the inferior pole of the patella and occurs due to an acute injury and must be differentiated from Sinding-Larsen-Johansson syndrome. The sleeve fracture includes an avulsion of a small bony fragment from the inferior pole of the patella with a large articular sleeve off of the bony patella. This injury occurs between the ages of 8 and 12.[55] The mechanism of injury is usually from tensile load of the patella with forceful contraction of the quadriceps against resistance.

The clinical presentation is usually one of significant pain with a large hemarthrosis of the knee. Full extension and straight-leg raising are difficult and the patella is usually high-riding. Radiographs, in particular a lateral radiograph, show a small bony fragment that tears away from the inferior pole of the patella as well as patella alta (**Fig. 4**). Treatment of patella sleeve fractures is operative with careful reapproximation of the sleeve of cartilage. Modified tension-band wiring around screws or Kirschner wires helps centralize and reduce the fragment.[55] Immobilization for a short time (3 to 4 weeks) followed by mobilization is required.

Tibial tuberosity fracture
Avulsion fractures of the tibial tuberosity are uncommon but tend occur in 13-to 16-year-old boys involved in a leaping activity. The male-to-female ratio is approximately 5:1 and bilateral fractures have been reported.[56–59] Physical examination findings depend on

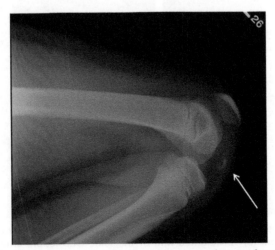

Fig. 4. Patellar sleeve fracture on lateral radiograph; arrow denotes fracture.

the magnitude and severity of the injury. The joint is usually held at 20° to 40°, there is a hemarthrosis, and the amount of patella alta is dependent on the displacement of the tubercle. Plain radiographs, especially the lateral view, confirm the diagnosis (**Fig. 5**).

If the fracture is minimally or nondisplaced, a cylinder cast for 3 to 4 weeks can be used to allow for healing of the fracture. In cases of displaced fractures, open reduction and internal fixation of the fracture are necessary to achieve anatomic alignment and restore the quadriceps-patellar mechanism. As with other fractures, the tibial tuberosity fracture can extend into the physis of the proximal tibia and careful postoperative follow-up should monitor for signs of genu recurvatum or other angular deformities.

Tibial spine (intercondylar eminence)

Fractures of the tibial spine occur because of a chondroepiphyseal avulsion of the ACL insertion on the tibial eminence. Tibial spine fractures were once thought the pediatric equivalent of midsubstance ACL tears in adults, although recent evidence suggests that ACL tears in children are increasing[60] and the tibial spine fracture in adults is more common than previously thought.[61] Historically, the most common mechanism has been a fall from a bicycle, but an upsurge in participation in sports has led to an increase in tibial spine fractures.

Patients typically present with a painful swollen knee and are often unable to bear weight. Lateral radiographs are often diagnostic, although MRI can be useful to identify meniscal entrapment or tears (**Fig. 6**).[62,63] Grading of a tibial spine fracture is based on the Meyers and McKeever classification: grade I—nondisplaced, grade II—posteriorly hinged, and grade III—completely displaced.[64] Treatment is based on grading, with grade I, some grade II without laxity, and grade II or III fractures that are successfully reduced with closed maneuvers treated with cast immobilization. Grade II fractures with laxity and grade III fractures that are not reducible are treated surgically. Arthoscopic or open reduction with internal fixation of the tibial spine is performed using suture or cannulated screws.[65–67] Patients are placed in a postoperative hinged knee brace and early initiation of physical therapy is done. Functional ACL bracing can be used if there is residual knee laxity.

Cruciate Ligament Injury

Anterior cruciate

ACL injuries are unfortunately seen with increasing frequency and severity.[60] Stanitski and colleagues[68] reported in 70 children and adolescents with acute traumatic hemarthrosis that 47% of those ages 7 to 12 and 65% of those ages 13 to 18 had suffered a torn ACL. The mechanism of injury is similar to that of adults, with a deceleration of the patient while planting a foot and turning in the opposite direction. The

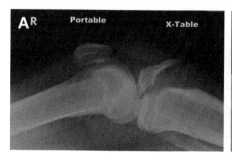
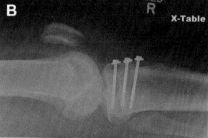

Fig. 5. (*A*) Tibial tuberosity fracture (Salter-Harris IV). (*B*) After open reduction and internal fixation with 3 screws.

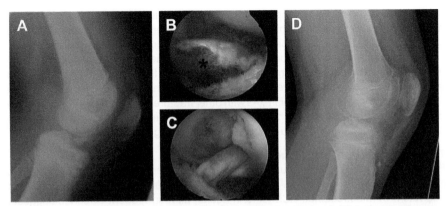

Fig. 6. (*A*) Displaced tibial spine fracture shown on lateral radiograph (*B*) Arthroscopic exposure of the tibial spine fracture with the fragment (*asterisk*) elevated off the tibial plateau. (*C*) Arthroscopic reduction of the tibial spine fracture with sutures around the ACL. (*D*) Anatomically reduced tibial spine fracture after fixation.

resultant valgus stress causes anterior displacement of the tibia and injury to the ligament. Patients usually reported feeling or hearing a pop at the time and are usually unable to continue the activity. A large hemarthrosis usually develops, which limits range of motion. The Lachman test is most useful for clinical assessment, although an MRI is diagnostic (**Fig. 7**).

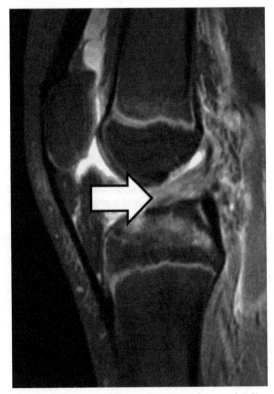

Fig. 7. MRI image of torn ACL; arrow denotes location of normal ACL.

The ligament may be fully or partially torn, and treatment options depend on the severity of the injury. Nonoperative management of partial tears may be successful in younger patients, those with a negative pivot shift test, and those with less than 50% of the ligament ruptured.[69] Depending on age of the patient and the potential growth remaining in the distal femoral and proximal tibial physis, treatment of can consistent of conservative or operative measures. Bracing and conservative management can be used as the primary treatment option, with a goal of stabilizing the patient until close to skeletal maturity. This may result, however, in decreased activity level, continued instability, or an increased rate of intra-articular damage, which may have long-term negative consequences in the development of degenerative joint disease.[70–73]

Adolescents close to the end of growth or who are skeletally mature should undergo contemporary adult ACL reconstruction techniques.[74] In those patients who are pre-pubescent, physeal-sparing techniques have been described that include the two most used techniques: an intra-articular extra-articular reconstruction using iliotibial band and an all-epiphyseal technique using bone tunnels.[75,76] Patients are placed in a brace postoperatively and physical therapy is initiated quickly.

Posterior cruciate

PCL injuries are rare, with most cases case reports of a bony avulsion injury. The mechanism of injury is oftentimes an anterior blow to the tibia of a flexed knee. Clinical presentation is similar to the ACL with a large tense hemarthrosis and difficulty with range of motion. Lateral radiographs are often helpful to show bony avulsions, and MRI can be used to confirm the diagnosis. Treatment is usually nonoperative, unless there is significant displacement of the bony avulsion or gross instability due to a complete rupture. Kocher and colleagues[77] recently described the largest series of PCL injuries in children and adolescents, in which 57% underwent operative intervention.

Collateral Ligament Injury

Isolated injury to the MCL in children is uncommon, and injury to the LCL is even more rare.[78] Collateral ligament injuries are graded as grades I to III. Grade I injuries are characterized by pain and tenderness along the course of the ligament without instability. Grade II injuries are associated with ligamentous laxity and represent partial tears, which present with increased laxity with varus or valgus force but a discrete endpoint. Grade II injuries are complete tears with no discernable endpoint to varus or valgus force.

Radiographs may demonstrate a distal cortical fleck fragment with either medial or LCL injuries; proximal or midsubstance injuries are uncommon. The injuries generally respond well to nonoperative treatment with a period of immobilization in a hinged knee brace for 6 weeks followed by physical therapy. Care must be taken to ensure that there is no concomitant cruciate ligament injury or multiplanar instability. In those settings, operative repair of the collateral ligaments should be considered. Sankar and colleagues[79] reported on a small series of pediatric ACL/MCL injuries treated with nonoperative management of a grade II or grade III MCL with ACL reconstruction. At 5 years, all patients had stable knees and returned to sports similar to adult injury patterns.

Meniscal Injury

The meniscus can be torn acutely with a sudden twisting injury to the knee or can occur in association with a prolonged degenerative process, such as an ACL-deficient knee.[72] Classic signs of meniscal injury include locking and giving way, although these, along with the McMurray sign, often are absent in children. It is, therefore, not uncommon that meniscal injuries, in particular injuries to a discoid meniscus, often go undiagnosed for long periods of time. MRI may be useful in the diagnosis of these injuries.

The treatment of meniscal injuries is still somewhat controversial. Asymptomatic discoid meniscus is treated with observation. Partial and total meniscectomy have been performed in children, although an increase in the contact stresses of the knee and poor long-term outcomes have not made this a favorable procedure.[20,22] Symptomatic meniscal tears are treated with meniscal repair using arthroscopic inside-out, outside-in, or all-inside techniques. Symptomatic discoid meniscus is treated with saucerization of the meniscus and repair to the capsule as indicated.

Patellofemoral Injury

Patellofemoral instability is one of the more common conditions seen around the knee in pediatric and adolescent patients.[80,81] Most patella dislocations or subluxations occur in the lateral direction. Medial dislocations or subluxations are exceedingly rare and usually a result of a direct blow or iatrogenic surgical result.[82] Patients usually report a feeling of the knee giving way, with the possibility of either a spontaneous or manual reduction. There may be a large effusion and usually significant pain medially around the patella. The Q-angle should be assessed and patellar apprehension test used if clinically indicated. Radiographs, if obtained, should include the anteroposterior, lateral, and Merchant views. The lateral view is important to assess for patella alta and trochlea dysplasia.[83,84] If indicated, MRI can be useful to detect chondral injury, osteochondral fractures, or large medial patellar stabilizer defects.

Nonoperative treatment, with closed reduction and immobilization followed by rehabilitation, bracing, and strengthening, is the standard of treatment of the majority of first-time dislocations.[85–88] Those dislocations that have a concomitant chondral injury, osteochondral fracture, or significant medial patellar stabilizer defect may be candidates for early operative intervention.[81] Several studies have shown, however, that almost half of patients have recurrent instability or pain.[81,89,90] The largest risk factor seems to be skeletally immature patients with trochlear dysplasia.[91]

Operative intervention for patella instability in children and adolescents is constrained by the open physes and well over 100 procedures have been described for the treatment. The chondral injury of the knee is addressed first with the next goal re-establishing the balance of forces of the patella.[92] Techniques include releasing tight lateral structures, restoring medial restraints by reefing or medial patellofemoral ligament reconstruction, and improving anatomic alignment.[93] Distal realignment procedures are often reserved until skeletal maturity. Recently, the use of medial patellofemoral ligament reconstruction in skeletally immature patients has been gaining favor.[94]

REFERENCES

1. Rosenblatt RA, Cherkin DC, Schneeweiss R, et al. The content of ambulatory medical care in the United States. An interspecialty comparison. N Engl J Med 1983;309(15):892–7.
2. Houghton KM. Review for the generalist: evaluation of pediatric hip pain. Pediatr Rheumatol Online J 2009;7:10.
3. Ahmad CS, McCarthy M, Gomez JA, et al. The moving patellar apprehension test for lateral patellar instability. Am J Sports Med 2009;37(4):791–6.

4. Rubinstein RA Jr, Shelbourne KD, McCarroll JR, et al. The accuracy of the clinical examination in the setting of posterior cruciate ligament injuries. Am J Sports Med 1994;22(4):550–7.
5. Donaldson WF 3rd, Warren RF, Wickiewicz T. A comparison of acute anterior cruciate ligament examinations. Initial versus examination under anesthesia. Am J Sports Med 1985;13(1):5–10.
6. Jonsson T, Althoff B, Peterson L, et al. Clinical diagnosis of ruptures of the anterior cruciate ligament: a comparative study of the Lachman test and the anterior drawer sign. Am J Sports Med 1982;10(2):100–2.
7. Mitsou A, Vallianatos P. Clinical diagnosis of ruptures of the anterior cruciate ligament: a comparison between the Lachman test and the anterior drawer sign. Injury 1988;19(6):427–8.
8. Katz JW, Fingeroth RJ. The diagnostic accuracy of ruptures of the anterior cruciate ligament comparing the Lachman test, the anterior drawer sign, and the pivot shift test in acute and chronic knee injuries. Am J Sports Med 1986; 14(1):88–91.
9. Kim SJ, Kim HK. Reliability of the anterior drawer test, the pivot shift test, and the Lachman test. Clin Orthop Relat Res 1995;(317):237–42.
10. Torg JS, Conrad W, Kalen V. Clinical diagnosis of anterior cruciate ligament instability in the athlete. Am J Sports Med 1976;4(2):84–93.
11. Marshall JL, Rubin RM. Knee ligament injuries—a diagnostic and therapeutic approach. Orthop Clin North Am 1977;8(3):641–68.
12. Fowler PJ, Lubliner JA. The predictive value of five clinical signs in the evaluation of meniscal pathology. Arthroscopy 1989;5(3):184–6.
13. Kurosaka M, Yagi M, Yoshiya S, et al. Efficacy of the axially loaded pivot shift test for the diagnosis of a meniscal tear. Int Orthop 1999;23(5):271–4.
14. McMurray TP. The semilunar cartilages. Br J Surg 1942;29:407–14.
15. Bauer SJ, Hollander JE, Fuchs SH, et al. A clinical decision rule in the evaluation of acute knee injuries. J Emerg Med 1995;13(5):611–5.
16. Rivara FP, Parish RA, Mueller BA. Extremity injuries in children: predictive value of clinical findings. Pediatrics 1986;78(5):803–7.
17. Seaberg DC, Jackson R. Clinical decision rule for knee radiographs. Am J Emerg Med 1994;12(5):541–3.
18. Weber JE, Jackson RE, Peacock WF, et al. Clinical decision rules discriminate between fractures and nonfractures in acute isolated knee trauma. Ann Emerg Med 1995;26(4):429–33.
19. Seaberg DC, Yealy DM, Lukens T, et al. Multicenter comparison of two clinical decision rules for the use of radiography in acute, high-risk knee injuries. Ann Emerg Med 1998;32(1):8–13.
20. Deanehan JK, Nigrovic PA, Milewski MD, et al. Synovial fluid findings in children with knee monoarthritis in lyme disease endemic areas. Pediatr Emerg Care 2014;30(1):16–9.
21. Milewski MD, Cruz AI Jr, Miller CP, et al. Lyme arthritis in children presenting with joint effusions. J Bone Joint Surg Am 2011;93(3):252–60.
22. Thompson A, Mannix R, Bachur R. Acute pediatric monoarticular arthritis: distinguishing lyme arthritis from other etiologies. Pediatrics 2009;123(3):959–65.
23. Ehrenborg G. The Osgood-Schlatter lesion. A clinical study of 170 cases. Acta Chir Scand 1962;124:89–105.
24. Wall EJ. Osgood-schlatter disease: practical treatment for a self-limiting condition. Phys Sportsmed 1998;26(3):29–34.

25. Kujala UM, Kvist M, Heinonen O. Osgood-Schlatter's disease in adolescent athletes. Retrospective study of incidence and duration. Am J Sports Med 1985;13(4):236–41.
26. Bloom OJ, Mackler L, Barbee J. Clinical inquiries. What is the best treatment for Osgood-Schlatter disease? J Fam Pract 2004;53(2):153–6.
27. Grass AL. Treatment of Osgood-Schlatter injury. JAMA 1978;240(3):212–3.
28. Levine J, Kashyap S. A new conservative treatment of Osgood-Schlatter disease. Clin Orthop Relat Res 1981;(158):126–8.
29. Soren A. Treatment of Osgood-Schlatter disease. Am J Orthop Surg 1968; 10(3):70–1.
30. Nierenberg G, Falah M, Keren Y, et al. Surgical treatment of residual osgood-schlatter disease in young adults: role of the mobile osseous fragment. Orthopedics 2011;34(3):176.
31. Orava S, Malinen L, Karpakka J, et al. Results of surgical treatment of unresolved Osgood-Schlatter lesion. Ann Chir Gynaecol 2000;89(4):298–302.
32. Medlar RC, Lyne ED. Sinding-Larsen-Johansson disease. Its etiology and natural history. J Bone Joint Surg Am 1978;60(8):1113–6.
33. Dupont JY. Synovial plicae of the knee. Controversies and review. Clin Sports Med 1997;16(1):87–122.
34. Patel D. Plica as a cause of anterior knee pain. Orthop Clin North Am 1986; 17(2):273–7.
35. Amatuzzi MM, Fazzi A, Varella MH. Pathologic synovial plica of the knee. Results of conservative treatment. Am J Sports Med 1990;18(5):466–9.
36. Hardaker WT, Whipple TL, Bassett FH 3rd. Diagnosis and treatment of the plica syndrome of the knee. J Bone Joint Surg Am 1980;62(2):221–5.
37. Mital MA, Hayden J. Pain in the knee in children: the medial plica shelf syndrome. Orthop Clin North Am 1979;10(3):713–22.
38. Dorchak JD, Barrack RL, Kneisl JS, et al. Arthroscopic treatment of symptomatic synovial plica of the knee. Long-term followup. Am J Sports Med 1991;19(5): 503–7.
39. Johnson DP, Eastwood DM, Witherow PJ. Symptomatic synovial plicae of the knee. J Bone Joint Surg Am 1993;75(10):1485–96.
40. Cahill BR. Osteochondritis dissecans of the knee: treatment of juvenile and adult forms. J Am Acad Orthop Surg 1995;3(4):237–47.
41. Glancy GL. Juvenile osteochondritis dissecans. Am J Knee Surg 1999;12(2): 120–4.
42. Green WT, Banks HH. Osteochondritis dissecans in children. J Bone Joint Surg Am 1953;35-A(1):26–47 passim.
43. Kocher MS, Tucker R, Ganley TJ, et al. Management of osteochondritis dissecans of the knee: current concepts review. Am J Sports Med 2006;34(7): 1181–91.
44. Wall EJ, Vourazeris J, Myer GD, et al. The healing potential of stable juvenile osteochondritis dissecans knee lesions. J Bone Joint Surg Am 2008;90(12): 2655–64.
45. Aglietti P, Buzzi R, Bassi PB, et al. Arthroscopic drilling in juvenile osteochondritis dissecans of the medial femoral condyle. Arthroscopy 1994;10(3):286–91.
46. Aglietti P, Ciardullo A, Giron F, et al. Results of arthroscopic excision of the fragment in the treatment of osteochondritis dissecans of the knee. Arthroscopy 2001;17(7):741–6.
47. Anderson AF, Richards DB, Pagnani MJ, et al. Antegrade drilling for osteochondritis dissecans of the knee. Arthroscopy 1997;13(3):319–24.

48. Johnson LL, Uitvlugt G, Austin MD, et al. Osteochondritis dissecans of the knee: arthroscopic compression screw fixation. Arthroscopy 1990;6(3):179–89.
49. Kocher MS, Micheli LJ, Yaniv M, et al. Functional and radiographic outcome of juvenile osteochondritis dissecans of the knee treated with transarticular arthroscopic drilling. Am J Sports Med 2001;29(5):562–6.
50. Navarro R, Cohen M, Filho MC, et al. The arthroscopic treatment of osteochondritis dissecans of the knee with autologous bone sticks. Arthroscopy 2002; 18(8):840–4.
51. Peterson L, Minas T, Brittberg M, et al. Treatment of osteochondritis dissecans of the knee with autologous chondrocyte transplantation: results at two to ten years. J Bone Joint Surg Am 2003;85-A(Suppl 2):17–24.
52. Steadman JR, Briggs KK, Rodrigo JJ, et al. Outcomes of microfracture for traumatic chondral defects of the knee: average 11-year follow-up. Arthroscopy 2003;19(5):477–84.
53. Dai LY, Zhang WM. Fractures of the patella in children. Knee Surg Sports Traumatol Arthrosc 1999;7(4):243–5.
54. Bishay M. Sleeve fracture of upper pole of patella. J Bone Joint Surg Br 1991; 73(2):339.
55. Houghton GR, Ackroyd CE. Sleeve fractures of the patella in children: a report of three cases. J Bone Joint Surg Br 1979;61-B(2):165–8.
56. Bolesta MJ, Fitch RD. Tibial tubercle avulsions. J Pediatr Orthop 1986;6(2): 186–92.
57. Lepse PS, McCarthy RE, McCullough FL. Simultaneous bilateral avulsion fracture of the tibial tuberosity. A case report. Clin Orthop Relat Res 1988;(229): 232–5.
58. Mirbey J, Besancenot J, Chambers RT, et al. Avulsion fractures of the tibial tuberosity in the adolescent athlete. Risk factors, mechanism of injury, and treatment. Am J Sports Med 1988;16(4):336–40.
59. Ogden JA, Tross RB, Murphy MJ. Fractures of the tibial tuberosity in adolescents. J Bone Joint Surg Am 1980;62(2):205–15.
60. Shea KG, Pfeiffer R, Wang JH, et al. Anterior cruciate ligament injury in pediatric and adolescent soccer players: an analysis of insurance data. J Pediatr Orthop 2004;24(6):623–8.
61. Kieser DC, Gwynne-Jones D, Dreyer S. Displaced tibial intercondylar eminence fractures. J Orthop Surg (Hong Kong) 2011;19(3):292–6.
62. Ishibashi Y, Tsuda E, Sasaki T, et al. Magnetic resonance imaging aids in detecting concomitant injuries in patients with tibial spine fractures. Clin Orthop Relat Res 2005;(434):207–12.
63. Kocher MS, Micheli LJ, Gerbino P, et al. Tibial eminence fractures in children: prevalence of meniscal entrapment. Am J Sports Med 2003;31(3):404–7.
64. Meyers MH, McKeever FM. Fracture of the intercondylar eminence of the tibia. J Bone Joint Surg Am 1959;41-A(2):209–20 [discussion: 220–2].
65. Hapa O, Barber FA, Suner G, et al. Biomechanical comparison of tibial eminence fracture fixation with high-strength suture, EndoButton, and suture anchor. Arthroscopy 2012;28(5):681–7.
66. Johnson DL, Durbin TC. Physeal-sparing tibial eminence fracture fixation with a headless compression screw. Orthopedics 2012;35(7):604–8.
67. Lehman RA Jr, Murphy KP, Machen MS, et al. Modified arthroscopic suture fixation of a displaced tibial eminence fracture. Arthroscopy 2003;19(2):E6.
68. Stanitski CL, Harvell JC, Fu F. Observations on acute knee hemarthrosis in children and adolescents. J Pediatr Orthop 1993;13(4):506–10.

69. Kocher MS, Micheli LJ, Zurakowski D, et al. Partial tears of the anterior cruciate ligament in children and adolescents. Am J Sports Med 2002;30(5): 697–703.

70. Graf BK, Lange RH, Fujisaki CK, et al. Anterior cruciate ligament tears in skeletally immature patients: meniscal pathology at presentation and after attempted conservative treatment. Arthroscopy 1992;8(2):229–33.

71. Janarv PM, Nystrom A, Werner S, et al. Anterior cruciate ligament injuries in skeletally immature patients. J Pediatr Orthop 1996;16(5):673–7.

72. Millett PJ, Willis AA, Warren RF. Associated injuries in pediatric and adolescent anterior cruciate ligament tears: does a delay in treatment increase the risk of meniscal tear? Arthroscopy 2002;18(9):955–9.

73. Mizuta H, Kubota K, Shiraishi M, et al. The conservative treatment of complete tears of the anterior cruciate ligament in skeletally immature patients. J Bone Joint Surg Br 1995;77(6):890–4.

74. Kocher MS, Smith JT, Zoric BJ, et al. Transphyseal anterior cruciate ligament reconstruction in skeletally immature pubescent adolescents. J Bone Joint Surg Am 2007;89(12):2632–9.

75. Anderson AF. Transepiphyseal replacement of the anterior cruciate ligament using quadruple hamstring grafts in skeletally immature patients. J Bone Joint Surg Am 2004;86-A(Suppl 1(Pt 2)):201–9.

76. Kocher MS, Garg S, Micheli LJ. Physeal sparing reconstruction of the anterior cruciate ligament in skeletally immature prepubescent children and adolescents. J Bone Joint Surg Am 2005;87(11):2371–9.

77. Kocher MS, Shore B, Nasreddine AY, et al. Treatment of posterior cruciate ligament injuries in pediatric and adolescent patients. J Pediatr Orthop 2012;32(6): 553–60.

78. Bradley GW, Shives TC, Samuelson KM. Ligament injuries in the knees of children. J Bone Joint Surg Am 1979;61(4):588–91.

79. Sankar WN, Wells L, Sennett BJ, et al. Combined anterior cruciate ligament and medial collateral ligament injuries in adolescents. J Pediatr Orthop 2006;26(6): 733–6.

80. Nietosvaara Y, Aalto K, Kallio PE. Acute patellar dislocation in children: incidence and associated osteochondral fractures. J Pediatr Orthop 1994;14(4): 513–5.

81. Stefancin JJ, Parker RD. First-time traumatic patellar dislocation: a systematic review. Clin Orthop Relat Res 2007;455:93–101.

82. Hughston JC, Deese M. Medial subluxation of the patella as a complication of lateral retinacular release. Am J Sports Med 1988;16(4):383–8.

83. Dejour H, Walch G, Nove-Josserand L, et al. Factors of patellar instability: an anatomic radiographic study. Knee Surg Sports Traumatol Arthrosc 1994;2(1): 19–26.

84. Thevenin-Lemoine C, Ferrand M, Courvoisier A, et al. Is the Caton-Deschamps index a valuable ratio to investigate patellar height in children? J Bone Joint Surg Am 2011;93(8):e35.

85. Buchner M, Baudendistel B, Sabo D, et al. Acute traumatic primary patellar dislocation: long-term results comparing conservative and surgical treatment. Clin J Sport Med 2005;15(2):62–6.

86. Cash JD, Hughston JC. Treatment of acute patellar dislocation. Am J Sports Med 1988;16(3):244–9.

87. Larsen E, Lauridsen F. Results of conservative treatment of patellar dislocations. Acta Orthop Belg 1982;48(3):455–62.

88. Palmu S, Kallio PE, Donell ST, et al. Acute patellar dislocation in children and adolescents: a randomized clinical trial. J Bone Joint Surg Am 2008;90(3): 463–70.

89. Cofield RH, Bryan RS. Acute dislocation of the patella: results of conservative treatment. J Trauma 1977;17(7):526–31.

90. Hawkins RJ, Bell RH, Anisette G. Acute patellar dislocations. The natural history. Am J Sports Med 1986;14(2):117–20.

91. Lewallen LW, McIntosh AL, Dahm DL. Predictors of recurrent instability after acute patellofemoral dislocation in pediatric and adolescent patients. Am J Sports Med 2013;41(3):575–81.

92. Stanitski CL, Paletta GA Jr. Articular cartilage injury with acute patellar dislocation in adolescents. Arthroscopic and radiographic correlation. Am J Sports Med 1998;26(1):52–5.

93. Stanitski CL. Patellar instability in the school age athlete. Instr Course Lect 1998; 47:345–50.

94. Deie M, Ochi M, Sumen Y, et al. Reconstruction of the medial patellofemoral ligament for the treatment of habitual or recurrent dislocation of the patella in children. J Bone Joint Surg Br 2003;85(6):887–90.

Lower Extremity Rotational and Angular Issues in Children

James F. Mooney III, MD

KEYWORDS

- Angular deformity • Rotational deformity • Femoral anteversion • Tibial torsion

KEY POINTS

- There is a wide range of normal lower extremity positioning in growing children.
- Angular and rotational status in children tends to follow standard developmental pathways over time.
- Little or no intervention, beyond reassurance, is necessary for most patients, and their parents, who present with concerns regarding rotational or angular issues in children.

INTRODUCTION/OVERVIEW

Parental questions and concerns regarding lower extremity rotational and angular status are some of the most common musculoskeletal issues facing primary care physicians and pediatric orthopedic surgeons.[1] As such, it is important that all physicians providing care for children have a thorough understanding of appropriate methods of examination and of the natural history of these physical findings. In most patients, the natural history is benign, with self-resolution without the necessity of any active treatment as the general rule. However, there are rare patients who require further evaluation, and in some cases orthopedic management, to reach the end of skeletal development and growth with a normal rotational and/or angular profile of the lower extremities.

THE MUSCULOSKELETAL EVALUATION/PHYSICAL EXAMINATION

An appropriate musculoskeletal evaluation in children includes both a comprehensive history and physical examination. The parents should be questioned regarding birth history, issues during pregnancy, development, and attainment of motor milestones.

Disclosure: None.
Department of Orthopaedic Surgery, Medical University of South Carolina, 96 Jonathan Lucas Street, CSB708, Charleston, SC 29425, USA
E-mail address: jfm3md@aol.com

Pediatr Clin N Am 61 (2014) 1175–1183
http://dx.doi.org/10.1016/j.pcl.2014.08.006
0031-3955/14/$ – see front matter © 2014 Elsevier Inc. All rights reserved.

In addition, it is important to determine whether there is any family history of orthopedic or musculoskeletal disorders, particularly those that may cause pathologic rotational or angular deformities. In addition, it is valuable to ascertain whether the perceived abnormality is affecting the child's function or development in any way, such as causing gait problems, shoe wear issues, or tripping/falling. Overall, it is imperative to begin to differentiate those patients who are in the wide range of normal variants from those with significant developmental or structural abnormalities. Most patients are within the wide range of normal, but it is necessary to be aware of the possibility of true disorder. Children with significantly abnormal rotational or angular deformities, in conjunction with apparent positive familial or development history, should be referred for specialized musculoskeletal evaluation.

In addition to the patient history, it is essential that a detailed, but focused, musculoskeletal physical examination be performed on all patients with parental concerns. The examination should be performed in a standardized fashion, and should address all sites of potential abnormality. It is important that all primary care physicians taking care of children are capable of performing this examination, and attainment of this skill set must be part of any primary care training program. It is not acceptable simply to refer all musculoskeletal evaluations and questions to a specialist, because most of these parental issues and concerns are of a benign nature, are part of normal development, and require little more than knowledgeable reassurance.

The musculoskeletal examination does not need to be time consuming or lengthy, but does need to be thorough. A complete examination requires evaluation of the static and dynamic status of the lower limbs. It is important to look at the overall position of the limbs while the child is at rest, and, if the child has reached walking age, during standing and gait. The child must be undressed, or at least placed in a gown or disposable shorts to perform a proper examination (**Fig. 1**). Watching the child walk around the room may be acceptable, but with older or bigger children it may be best to view patients while they are walking away from and toward the examiner in a hallway or corridor. In addition, the general overview should include review of height and weight, stature, skin condition or lesions, limb girth, and appropriateness of development for chronologic age. All normal and abnormal findings should be documented in the medical record.

Staheli and colleagues[2] described and elucidated the concept of the child's rotational profile in 1985. These investigators evaluated 1000 normal children and adults, assessing lower extremity passive range of motion and rotational positioning of the

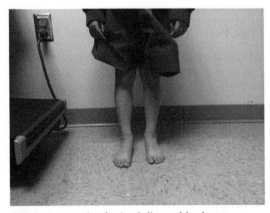

Fig. 1. A child standing in appropriately sized disposable shorts.

lower extremities. The data generated provide the largest single assessment of these issues, and constitutes what the clinicians consider to be normal values to this day. All components of this profile should be evaluated as part of the musculoskeletal examination. The components include external and internal rotation of the hips (assessing femoral version), thigh-foot axis (tibial torsion) (**Fig. 2**), transmalleolar angle, and foot progression angle with gait. Addressing another aspect of lower extremity rotation, Smith, Bleck and colleagues[3] promoted the concept of the heel bisector, which is useful in assessing rotation of the foot secondary to foot deformity. Although specifics of foot deformity and the heel bisector were not part of the original study by Staheli and colleagues,[2] it should be part of the general evaluation of a patient seen for rotational concerns.

The static or nonambulatory portion of the examination evaluating the child's rotational profile ideally should be performed with the patient prone (**Fig. 3**). This position provides the best assessment of lower extremity rotation, and allows the physician to view both limbs simultaneously. Sometimes this is a challenge in young patients because of agitation, and, with practice, a high-quality examination can be done with the patient supine, reclining slightly in the parent's lap. Visualization of the patient while walking is necessary to determine dynamic rotation during gait, and to assess the patient's foot progression angle. Patients who intoe during the stance phase of gait are considered to have negative foot progression angles, whereas those who out-toe have positive values.

The review of lower extremity angulation is done best with the patient standing, but can be assessed fairly well while sitting in those children unable or unwilling to stand. It is important to view the child while the patient is standing, both from the front and from the rear, to gain the best view of lower extremity limb angulation during weight bearing. Again, it is essential that the child be placed in a gown, shorts, or some other nonobstructive clothing to perform an adequate lower extremity evaluation.

SPECIFIC ISSUES
Intoeing/Out-toeing

Rotational issues in children, specifically intoeing and out-toeing, are among the most common musculoskeletal issues facing the primary care physician in office practice. It is important to know that most rotational issues are self-limiting, and require no active treatment.[4] Parental concerns regarding intoeing seem to far outnumber those regarding out-toeing in clinical practice. The possible sources of intoeing are femoral

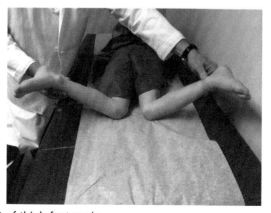

Fig. 2. Assessment of thigh-foot angle.

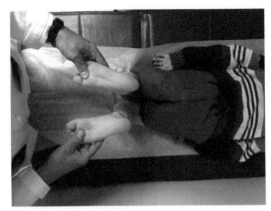

Fig. 3. A patient lying prone for examination of internal rotation of the hips.

anteversion, internal tibial torsion, and metatarsus adductus. Patients often present with intoeing secondary to a combination of these causes.

Femoral Anteversion

Femoral anteversion is the most common cause of perceived abnormal intoeing in childhood.[4] Version, or torsion, of the femoral neck is the angle between the axis of the femoral neck and the transverse axis of the knee. More simply, it is the angle that the femoral neck extends anteriorly from the shaft of the femur. This angle sets the amount of active and passive range of rotation at the hip. Neonates have an average of 40° of anteversion. This angle generally decreases, without intervention, to an average adult level of 15° by approximately 8 or 9 years of age.

Intoeing secondary to increased anteversion tends to be more common in girls than in boys, and is usually symmetric. Children with increased anteversion often run with a circumduction gait because of the internal rotation at the hip, and the parents may note that the child W-sits rather than sitting cross-legged. Physical examination shows increased internal rotation at the hip versus external rotation, and the foot progression angle is negative.

The natural history of intoeing secondary to increased femoral anteversion is almost universally benign. As noted previously, the increased internal rotation resolves as the femoral anteversion changes up to 8 or 9 years of age, and no intervention is required. Special shoes, braces, and bars between the shoes have not been shown to have any positive effect, and there is evidence of negative psychological impact of the use of orthopedic shoes and braces later in life.[5,6] Admonishment against W-sitting is of no value, because that position is the position of comfort for the child, and is in no way detrimental to normal development. Contrary to generations of misinformation, W-sitting does not lead to, or promote, intoeing in children. Children stop sitting in this position when they are able to sit cross-legged more comfortably, and this occurs as the natural progression to a mature value of femoral anteversion occurs. The only intervention that changes the natural history is the use of surgical femoral derotational osteotomy, and the indications for such a procedure in a neurologically normal child are extremely limited. Osteotomy is reserved for those children more than 8 or 9 years of age with severe functional or cosmetic limitations secondary to retained femoral anteversion greater than 45° to 50° and greater than 80° of internal rotation at the hip on physical examination.

Out-toeing secondary to abnormal decrease in femoral anteversion is uncommon. Physical examination in such a child shows a marked decrease in expected internal rotation at the hip, and increased external rotation. Because this is an unusual rotational profile for a child, this finding generally requires further evaluation and possibly subspecialist referral. Although no physical abnormality is found in many cases, decreased femoral anteversion, or in some cases true femoral retroversion, may be associated with congenital abnormalities of the proximal femur or lower limb, or may predispose the patient to other functional issues involving the lower extremity.

Internal and External Tibial Torsion

Internal tibial torsion is a common cause of intoeing in children, and often is seen in combination with increased femoral anteversion. Physical examination is necessary to differentiate between the two causes, and those patients with internal tibial torsion show an internally rotated thigh-foot angle (**Fig. 4**) and negative foot progression angle. Most patients have symmetric, bilateral involvement, but in unilateral cases the left limb seems to be more commonly involved. The cause of internal tibial torsion is unclear, but it is thought to be secondary to intrauterine positioning in most cases.

Patients with increased internal tibial torsion may have concomitant bowing of the lower leg (genu varum), which is a common finding in children less than 3 years of age. The combination of bowing and internal rotation may make the deformities appear more severe, and the physician must take care to assess and document both deformities. Issues regarding the natural history of genu varum are discussed later.

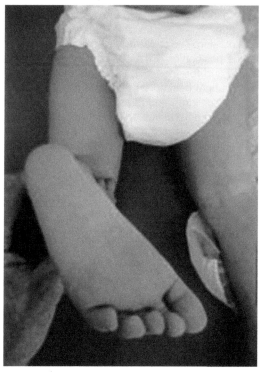

Fig. 4. Thigh-foot angle examination showing mild internal tibial torsion. (*From* Lincoln TL, Suen PW. Common rotational variations in children. J Am Acad Orthop Surg 2003;11(5):313; with permission.)

Most internal tibial torsion resolves spontaneously by the age of 4 to 5 years. For many years, patients were managed with special shoes and/or connecting bars (eg, Denis-Browne shoes and bars), which were worn at nights and during naps. Such items are not recommended at this time, because the rotation will resolve without intervention, and the shoes/bars do not provide any benefit to the deformity. Those few children who have persistent internal tibial torsion rarely have any significant issues, and residual torsion does not increase the risk of degenerative joint disease. Only those patients with severe residual deformity (>3 standard deviations beyond the mean) that causes severe functional or cosmetic abnormalities, and who are not expected to self-correct any further, are candidates for tibial derotational osteotomy.[4] In patients with internal torsion associated with neuromuscular disorders (eg, cerebral palsy, myelodysplasia), or in conjunction with other pathologic limb deformities (eg, clubfeet), tibial derotational osteotomy may be indicated more frequently.

In rare cases, a child presents with an out-toeing gait and examination is consistent with a diagnosis of external tibial torsion. These patients have positive foot progression angles, and externally rotated thigh/foot angles. Because tibial torsion tends to externally rotate up to the age of 4 to 5 years, preexisting external tibial torsion may increase. There is some evidence of an increased risk of patellofemoral pain and instability in patients with significant external tibial torsion. As such, those uncommon patients with severe external tibial torsion may require further evaluation by a pediatric orthopedic specialist and possibly surgical intervention.

Metatarsus Adductus

The third potential source of intoeing and lower extremity internal rotation deformity is metatarsus adductus (**Fig. 5**). Such children present with a C-shaped foot and parental complaints of intoeing. The cause of the deformity is unclear, but is most likely a function of intrauterine positioning. Physical examination shows a foot with medial deviation of the midfoot and forefoot, but with a neutral or slightly valgus hindfoot. There is no evidence of a tight heel cord or equinus hindfoot, and in most cases the deformity is flexible. Most children and infants with true metatarsus adductus have bilateral and fairly symmetric deformities.

Metatarsus adductus may be classified based on the amount of medial deviation as determined by the heel bisector angle, or by the flexibility of the deformity.[3] Further

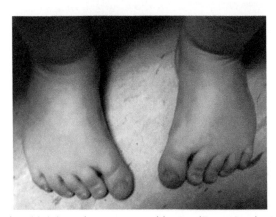

Fig. 5. Patient with mild, bilateral metatarsus adductus. (*From* Lincoln TL, Suen PW. Common rotational variations in children. J Am Acad Orthop Surg 2003;11(5):316; with permission.)

radiographic evaluation is unnecessary in young patients, and plain radiographs are not indicated except in rare cases.

Most metatarsus adductus deformities are mild and flexible, and generally resolve without intervention of any kind. Parental stretching programs may be instituted, but probably do not have any effect beyond simple reassurance. Ponseti and Becker[7] reported more than 300 patients with flexible metatarsus adductus, and in all cases there was improvement at 3 to 4 years of age without any formal treatment. Casting and special shoes are reserved for those patients with severe and rigid deformities, and these are a distinct minority of patients. Adjustable shoes have been shown to be as clinically effective, and more cost-effective, than serial casting programs for those rare patients requiring intervention.[8,9] Surgery is indicated only for those patients who fail casting for severe and rigid deformities, or who present late with deformities that affect shoe wear and function.

ANGULAR DEFORMITIES
Overview

Knee alignment in children changes during skeletal development, and tends to do so in a predictable pattern in most patients. Most children start with an element of genu varum (bowed legs), progress toward neutral alignment with growth, and then may develop significant genu valgum (knock knees) before returning to the common mild physiologic valgus alignment of the lower limb around 5 or 6 years of age.

Genu Varum

Bowed legs are a common concern of parents, grandparents, and other caregivers. A large percentage of pediatric patients develop, or are born with, some degree of genu varum, often in conjunction with physiologic internal tibial torsion.[10] The exact cause of this bowing is unclear, but because of its common nature, and because most cases resolve with time, this deformity is often described as physiologic bowing.

As noted, the exact cause of physiologic bowing is unclear. Multiple studies have documented the normal range of bowing for children during development. These norms seem to hold for children of multiple geographic and racial backgrounds. Salenius and Vankka, as well as Engel and Staheli, showed that pediatric knee alignment is initially 10° to 15° of varus (bowlegged) at birth, and reaches a neutral alignment by approximately 2 years of age. A more recent study of children in Turkey confirmed this natural history in that patient population.[11,12] In most cases, this bowing is bilateral and symmetric, and involves both the tibia and the distal femur. Intervention with orthotics, bracing, or connective bars is not indicated in most cases. Bowing that is of more concern, and for which further evaluation (radiographs, specialist consultation) may be indicated, includes that seen in patients with apparent unilateral bowing, evidence of associated endocrine abnormalities, or those patients who do not improve spontaneously by the age of 2 years.

Physical assessment of angular deformities, similar to examination of the patient's rotational profile, is best performed with the patient standing. Weight bearing accentuates the lower extremity angular status, and in most cases parents become concerned about this once the child begins to stand and walk. As with any examination of the lower extremities, it is important for the physician to look at the child with the legs uncovered by clothing, and to watch the child stand or walk. In addition, it is valuable to assess the patient's overall height and weight, and to document these on a growth chart.

Most patients with genu varum require no active treatment of any kind, because the natural history of this type of bowing is for the deformity to resolve spontaneously over time. The limbs progress back toward neutral and then to moderate valgus in most children. Bracing, special shoes, and inserts are not indicated, and have no effect on physiologic bowing. Reassurance should be the treatment of choice. Bracing or surgical intervention may be indicated in a small percentage of patients (eg, infantile Blount disease, skeletal dysplasias, bony manifestations of endocrine or renal abnormalities), but this is at the discretion of a pediatric orthopedic surgeon, possibly in conjunction with care of other pediatric specialists.

Genu Valgum

Genu valgum (knock knees) is a common finding in patents between the ages of 3 and 6 years. As noted previously, lower extremity angular development tends to move into a valgus alignment starting at approximately 3 years of age. At times, this valgus positioning appears severe, and may reach 20°. Families may have concerns about not only the alignment of the limb but the appearance of clumsiness and running pattern, as well as the effect that such positioning will have on the child's future development.

Salenius and Vankka showed that the maximum genu valgum during normal development was approximately 12° to 13°. However, higher levels of valgus are common, and most patients normalize without intervention. The child should be examined as for any musculoskeletal evaluation, and height and weight should be documented.

Radiographs and further specialty evaluation should be reserved for patients with severe deformities, particularly if the patient is greater than 5 to 6 years of age. Other indications for referral and/or radiographs include significant deviations from the norm for height or weight, unilateral or asymmetric deformity, or those patients in whom an endocrine abnormality or skeletal dysplasia is suspected.

No intervention beyond reassurance is indicated in most patients with genu valgum. Shoes, shoe inserts, connecting bars, and/or bracing have no role in these patients, despite their widespread use in the past. The natural history studies on this subject are clear as to the self-resolving and benign nature of genu valgum in most patients, as it is in genu varum. Surgical management is reserved for those patients who do not resolve spontaneously or who have extreme deformity.

SUMMARY

Parental concerns regarding rotational and angular deformities of the lower limbs in children are common. As such, it is important for the primary care provider to understand and master the basics of the lower extremity musculoskeletal examination. In addition, it is important for the primary care provider to understand the natural history of lower extremity rotational and angular development. However, the natural history is well documented, and is predictable in most cases. Most lower extremity rotational and angular issues resolve spontaneously with time, and as such require no intervention of any kind. Reassurance of the family is the only treatment indicated in almost all cases. In the rare patients with severe or unusual deformities, or in those patients who do not seem to follow the expected and predicted natural history, further evaluation or specialty referral may be indicated.

REFERENCES

1. Hsu EY, Schwend RM, Julia L. How many referrals to a pediatric orthopaedic hospital specialty clinic are primary care problems? J Pediatr Orthop 2012;32(7): 727–31.
2. Staheli LT, Corbett M, Wyss C, et al. Lower extremity rotational problems in children. J Bone Joint Surg Am 1985;67A:39–47.

3. Smith JT, Bleck EE, Gamble JG, et al. Simple method of documenting metatarsus adductus. J Pediatr Orthop 1991;11:679–80.
4. Lincoln TL, Suen PW. Common rotational variations in children. J Am Acad Orthop Surg 2003;11(5):312–20.
5. Wenger DR, Mauldin D, Speck G, et al. Corrective shoes and inserts as treatment for flexible flatfoot in infants and children. J Bone Joint Surg Am 1989;71:800–10.
6. Driano A, Staheli L, Staheli LT. Psychosocial development and corrective shoe-wear use in childhood. J Pediatr Orthop 1998;18(3):346–9.
7. Ponseti IV, Becker JR. Congenital metatarsus adductus: the results of treatment. J Bone Joint Surg Am 1966;48:702–11.
8. Allen WD, Weiner DS, Riley PM. The treatment of rigid metatarsus adductovarus with the use of a new hinged adjustable shoe orthosis. Foot Ankle 1993;14(8): 450–4.
9. Herzenberg JE, Burghardt RD. Treatment of resistant metatarsus adductus: prospective randomized trial of casting versus orthosis. J Orthop Sci 2014;8(2): 193–201.
10. Greene WB. Genu varum and genu valgum in children. Instructional course lectures. Chapter 15. Park Ridge (IL): AAOS; 1993. p. 151–9.
11. Heath CH, Staheli LT. Normal limits of knee angle in white children – genu varum and genu valgum. J Pediatr Orthop 1993;13(2):259–62.
12. Arazi M, Ogun TC, Memik R. Normal development of the tibiofemoral angle in children: a clinical study of 590 normal subjects fro 3 – 17 years of age. J Pediatr Orthop 2001;21(2):264–7.

Foot Pain in the Child and Adolescent

Amiethab Aiyer, MD, William Hennrikus, MD*

KEYWORDS

- Foot pain • Overuse syndromes • Osteonecrosis • Pediatric • Children

KEY POINTS

- There are multiple etiologies of foot pain in the child and adolescent.
- Most foot and ankle problems in the pediatric patient may be treated with a trial of conservative measures.
- Surgical intervention may be warranted in some patients in whom pain is refractory to nonoperative treatment.

INTRODUCTION

Pain in the foot and ankle of the child may arise from several different etiologies. In addition to understanding the developmental biology, anatomy, and biomechanics of the pediatric foot and ankle, a thorough history and physical examination are crucial to discerning a given cause of symptoms. In this review article, we aim to highlight some of the most common entities that we treat on a day-to-day basis. It is our goal for the reader to have a basic understanding of the pathomechanics behind some of these clinical problems to appropriately workup and optimally manage patients seen in this setting.

KOHLER'S DISEASE

Epidemiology

Kohler's disease was originally described at the beginning of the 20th century.[1] Most children who suffer from Kohler's disease are less than 10 years old. Bilateral cases may be seen in up to one fourth of cases.[1,2]

Pathophysiology

The primary blood supply to the navicular is via perforating branches of the dorsalis pedis. The intraosseous blood supply to the navicular leaves a central watershed at

Disclosures: The authors have relevant financial disclosures to report.
Department of Orthopaedic Surgery, Penn State College of Medicine, 30 Hope Drive, Hershey, PA 17033, USA
* Corresponding author.
E-mail address: wlh5k@hotmail.com

risk for avascular necrosis when blood flow is compromised. Most cases of Kohler's disease are idiopathic.[1]

Clinical Findings

There is often no specific attributable initiating event with Kohler's disease. Patients most often complain of midfoot pain that is exacerbated with weight bearing. On physical examination, the patient may be found to walk on the lateral border of the foot. Focal tenderness along the midfoot, in addition to swelling, may be seen.[2]

Imaging

On plain radiographs, sclerosis, fragmentation, and navicular flattening are seen. It is important to corroborate these findings with clinical ones, given that normal variants may have a similar appearance (**Fig. 1**).[1]

Treatment

The mainstay of management is nonoperative, with casting to help mitigate symptoms. Cast immobilization is used for 4 to 6 weeks.

Outcomes

The use of casting may help to increase the rate at which symptoms abate.[1] Although mild pain may be persist, most cases heal without long-term complications. Long-term

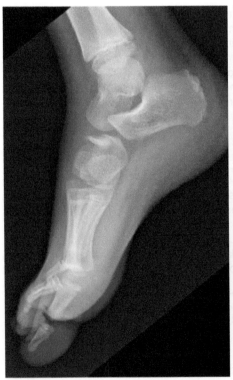
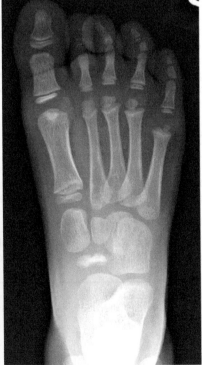

Fig. 1. Anteroposterior and lateral radiographs of Kohler's apophysitis of the tarsal navicular.

follow-up of these patients demonstrate that the navicular returns to its normal condition over time.[3,4]

SEVER'S DISEASE
Epidemiology

In the skeletally immature athlete, heel pain is a common complaint.[5,6] It is typically self-limited in nature and most commonly caused by calcaneal apophysitis or Sever's disease.[3,4] The condition has a reported incidence of 3.7 per 1000 and often affects children between 8 and 12 years of age. Achilles tendon contracture and deficiencies in shoe wear may lead to the development of Sever's disease.[2,7,8]

Pathophysiology

Although originally described as an inflammatory injury to the calcaneal apophysis, Sever's disease has been more recently attributed to mechanical overuse.[7] Ogden and colleagues[6] prospectively evaluated 14 patients with Sever's disease. The patients had magnetic resonance imaging (MRI) completed before and after treatment with immobilization was completed. Pretreatment MRI findings included trabecular bone bruising in the calcaneal metaphysis. Post-treatment MRIs demonstrated resolution of the metaphyseal findings, suggesting that this condition is likely related to increased metaphyseal stress as a result of biomechanical changes in a young, active child.

Clinical Findings

Those affected by Sever's disease commonly present with activity-dependent heel pain. Tenderness may be elicited over the posterior calcaneus at the level of the Achilles tendon insertion. The medial and lateral calcaneus may also by painful with compressive maneuvers.[2]

Imaging

Plain radiographs are of limited utility in the diagnosis of Sever's disease (**Fig. 2**). As demonstrated by Ogden and colleagues,[6] MRI may have more a diagnostic role in refractory cases. Findings on MRI include metaphyseal edema consistent with bone bruising (**Fig. 3**).

Treatment

Management is conservative in nature and based on the presence of symptoms. Analgesics, restricted weight bearing, or a short period of immobilization may be utilized.[2,6] Immobilization followed by physical therapy, with emphasis on heel cord

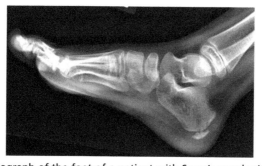

Fig. 2. Lateral radiograph of the foot of a patient with Sever's apophysitis.

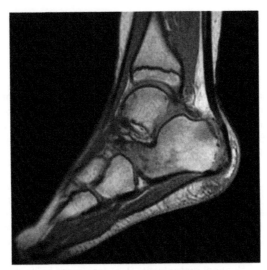

Fig. 3. MRI of Sever's apophysitis showing metaphyseal edema.

stretching, has been shown to be highly effective in allowing patients to return to pre-injury activity.[6,9] Use of plastizote heel supports and viscoelastic heel cups has been shown to be helpful in facilitating resolution of symptoms.[7]

Outcomes

Conservative measures are highly effective in allowing patients to get back to desired activities or sports.[6,10] Recurrence of symptoms is low.[7]

ISELIN'S DISEASE
Epidemiology

Iselin's disease was originally described in 1912. Although the reported prevalence is quite low, it is likely more common than previously thought. The condition often develops in young adolescents, as rapid growth occurs.[2,11] This coincides with the appearance of the proximal apophysis of the fifth metatarsal tuberosity (appears at approximately age 10 in females and approximately age 12 in males).[11]

Pathophysiology

Microtears in the tendinous attachment of the peroneus brevis at the base of the fifth metatarsal are thought to give rise to Iselin's disease.[2]

Clinical Findings

Patients with Iselin's disease have reproduction of symptoms with weight bearing and with activities in which inversional stresses are applied—running, jumping, and cutting maneuvers often lead to pain at the base of the fifth metatarsal. There may be a reported history of a prior ankle inversion injury.[12] On examination, pain may be elicited with palpation of an enlarged fifth metatarsal base (relative to the contralateral foot). Additionally, pain may be elicited with resisted plantarflexion and eversion.

Imaging

An oblique radiograph of the foot is most helpful; apophyseal enlargement may be identified. The apophysis has a shell shape and is found at the plantolateral aspect of the fifth metatarsal tuberosity (**Fig. 4**).[2] In contrast with fracture lines, the apophyseal line of the fifth metatarsal tuberosity lies parallel to the long axis of the metatarsal shaft. Fragmentation of this secondary center may be noted. Bone scans may be used when radiographs are normal and clinical suspicion is high; positive findings include increased signal uptake in the apophysis.[11]

Treatment

Iselin's disease may be managed conservatively and is noted to be a self-limiting condition. Some authors recommend use of short leg casts or walking boot during a brief period of immobilization. Slow return to activity after pain subsides is ideal; physical therapy may be used, with a focus on stretching and strengthening.

Outcomes

Symptom resolution may take months to years and coincides with apophyseal ossification. Although ossification occurs in most patients, symptomatic nonunion may be a rare long-term complication.[2,11]

RIGID FLATFOOT
Epidemiology

Tarsal coalitions are among the most common causes of rigid flat foot in the pediatric patient. The relative incidence of coalitions has been reported to be approximately 1%

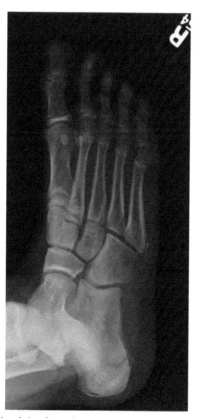

Fig. 4. Oblique radiograph of the foot demonstrating Iselin's apophyisitis.

to 2% of the population; talocalcaneal coalitions are more common than calcaneonavicular.[13] Bilateral cases are found in at least 50% of cases and males may be more frequently affected[13] The most common age for presentation is usually between 8 and 12 years old.[14]

Pathophysiology

Congenital tarsal coalitions result from deficiencies in mesenchymal segmentation when a patient is in utero. Such mesenchymal issues are inherited in an autosomal-dominant manner.[15] Although some authors believe that inheritance follows Mendelian genetics in a unifactorial fashion, others believe it to be more complicated. Plotkin's theory implicates multiple genes in the limb development pathway that would account for various sites of coalition development.[16] At birth, the coalition is present in a cartilaginous form; over time, ossification may lead to the development of symptoms. Calcaneonavicular coalitions present commonly at 8 to 12 years of age, whereas talocalcaneal coalitions usually present between 12 and 16 years of age.[17,18]

The presence of a coalition prevents internal rotation of the subtalar joint. This leads to compensatory forefoot abduction through the transverse tarsal joints and loss of the longitudinal arch. Subsequent peroneal spasm results in a spastic flatfoot.

In the setting of limited subtalar motion, the navicular attempts to improve dorsiflexion by overriding the talar head. Repetitive elevation of the dorsal capsule by this mechanism leads to a traction spur. This spur is thought to contribute to talar beak formation that is visualized on lateral radiographs.[19,20]

Clinical Findings

Patients with tarsal coalitions often present with pain during the second decade of life. Pain may be related to spasm of the peroneal tendons or the development of sinus tarsi syndromes. Additional complaints include difficulty with accommodation during gait as a result of compromised subtalar motion. This may lead to recurrent ankle sprains. On examination, the patient may have a rigid valgus hindfoot with compensatory forefoot abduction. Limited subtalar motion can be identified by asking patients to walk on the outer borders of their feet; patients with coalitions have difficulty with this maneuver.[15] Additionally, the longitudinal arch of the foot does not reconstitute with weight bearing or with toe rise.

Imaging

Initial radiographic evaluation is composed of standing anteroposterior (AP), lateral, and oblique views of the affected foot. It may difficult be to diagnose tarsal coalitions based on plain films because of the relative obliquity of the coalition itself, coalitions that are predominantly fibrocartilaginous, and superimposition of the osseous components themselves.[19] A lateral radiograph of talocalcaneal coalitions may demonstrate a C-sign, which is a composed of the talar dome and inferior aspect of the sustentaculum tali. Talar breaking may also be seen in either talocalcaneal or calcaneonavicular coalitions.[15] The oblique view is helpful identifying a calcaneonavicular coalition in most cases (**Fig. 5**). In the absence of a clear osseous bridge, stenosis of the calcaneonavicular joint, the presence of an elongated anterior calcaneal process, or irregularity of the cortices may serves as secondary indicators of a coalition.[15] Axial views may reveal the presence of a middle facet coalition, especially if is loss of the horizontal orientation of the middle facet.[15] Computed tomography (CT) can be obtained if plain radiographs are normal; narrowing of joint spaces and sclerosis may be indicative of the presence of a coalition (**Fig. 6**). MRI can be useful in delineating the presence of a fibrous or cartilaginous coalition and the presence of adjacent joint

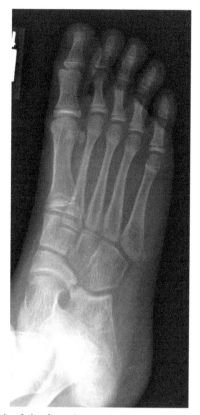

Fig. 5. Oblique radiograph of the foot demonstrating a calcaneal–navicular coalition.

arthritic changes (**Fig. 7**). Calcaneonavicular coalitions are best identified by sagittal and axial CT views. Coronal CT sections are best to visualize talocalcaneal coalitions.[15]

Treatment

Initial management is nonoperative in nature, with activity modification, functional bracing, and antiinflammatories for pain control.[15,21] Immobilization in a cast or walking boot may help to alleviate symptoms by limiting joint stresses.[15] Failure of conservative management to alleviate symptoms is an indication for operative intervention. Surgical options include resection or fusion. Resection of calcaneonavicular coalitions is often completed via an anterolateral approach, with coalition excision, followed by interposition of extensor digitorum brevis muscle or fat. When more than 50% of the joint surface was occupied by coalition, some authors have recommended isolated arthrodesis to maintain force transfer during gait.[22] A concern with isolated fusion is the potential for accelerated degeneration in other adjacent joints. The salvage procedure for failed resection procedures is a triple arthrodesis.[15]

Outcomes

Nonoperative measures have good outcomes in patients without evidence of joint compromise.[21,23] When nonoperative measures fail to alleviate pain, surgical resection is indicated. Success has been found with resection of talocalcaneal coalitions

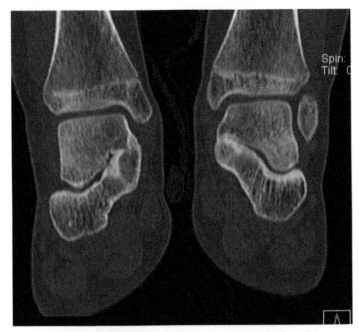

Fig. 6. Axial CT of bilateral feet demonstrating large talocalcaneal coalitions.

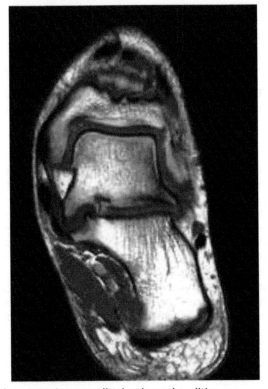

Fig. 7. Axial MRI demonstrating a small talocalcaneal coalition.

that occupied less than one third of the subtalar joint.[24] Poor outcomes after resection have been associated with the presence of concomitant hindfoot valgus and coalition areas of more than 50% of the posterior facet.[25] Others have found that, despite the high surface areas of the coalition, good outcomes could still be obtained.

Use of extensor digitorum brevis muscle interpositional grafts in resection of calcaneonavicular coalitions has yielded good outcomes among pediatric patients. However, Mubarak and colleagues[14] found that use of extensor digitorum brevis muscle interpositional grafts leads to cosmetic concerns and shoe wear irritation as the result of a prominent calcaneocuboid joint. To address this issue, the authors recommend use of fat interposition.

ACCESSORY NAVICULAR
Epidemiology

The accessory navicular (AN) is the most common ossicle in the foot and was originally described in the early 1600s.[26] The reported incidence is between 2% and 14% with the most recent reports noted a 11.7% incidence in the general population.[26,27]

Pathophysiology

The AN develops posterior and medial to the navicular tuberosity. It forms congenitally from a secondary ossification center that does not fuse with the navicular bone.[28] It often takes a pyramidal shape, with an anterior base and a posterior apex. It is connected to the navicular proper through fibers of the posterior tibial tendon, fibrous, or fibrocartilaginous connections.[26]

Clinical Findings

Patients with AN may become symptomatic during adolescence subsequent to medial foot irritation from shoe wear. Complaints of pain and tenderness may be increased with weight bearing or recreational activities.[29] Although controversy exists regarding the association between AN and the flatfoot deformity, no studies have demonstrated a true relationship between the 2 entities.[26,30]

Imaging

Standard weight-bearing radiographs, including a 45° external oblique view can be used to evaluate a patient for the presence of AN (**Fig. 8**). The use of an external oblique radiograph helps to more clearly delineate the AN, which lies posteromedial to the navicular tuberosity. If radiographs seem to be normal but a high degree of suspicion exists, a bone scan can be used to identify AN. On the bone scan, the AN will have increased signal uptake. Alternatively, an MRI can be used to differentiate AN from an avulsion injury.[26]

Treatment

Initial management measures should be conservative, with attempts to decrease medial foot pain by adjusting shoe wear. This can be accomplished with wider shoes and activity modification. Antiinflammatories can be a useful adjunct to help mitigate pain. Failure of conservative measures is an indication for surgery. Multiple options exist from excision of the AN, posterior tibial tendon advancement, percutaneous drilling, and fusion of the AN to the tarsal navicular.[26]

Outcomes

Many studies document the efficacy of surgical intervention for symptomatic AN. Perhaps one of the most well-known procedures is the Kidner procedure, which

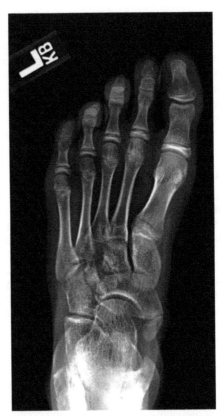

Fig. 8. External oblique radiograph of the foot demonstrating an accessory navicular.

was described in 1929. Other authors have challenged the original Kidner procedure, which was described to restore the line of pull of the posterior tibial tendon. In 1 study, no radiographic correction of the arch was seen with the Kidner procedure, leading the authors to believe that irritation of the posterior tibial tendon is the source of pain and dysfunction.[31] Others have shown that simple excision of the AN has led to symptomatic relief akin to the Kidner procedure; additionally, radiographic improvement of medial arch was seen in those treated conservatively or surgically, further questioning the association with pes planus.[32] Nakayama and colleagues[33] demonstrated good and excellent results with percutaneous drilling in type 2 ANs in young athletes. The authors note that this method is easy to complete, uses a limited incision, and minimizes complications. Arthrodesis of the AN versus the Kidner procedure was evaluated in 20 symptomatic patients. Patients who underwent the fusion procedure were found to have slightly improved American Orthopaedic Foot and Ankle Society scores.[34] Others have found fusion rates of approximately 80% coinciding with the ability for patients to return to sporting activities.[35]

FREIBERG'S DISEASE
Epidemiology

Freiberg's disease results from epiphyseal injury that leads to altered enchondral ossification.[36] Females are more commonly affected, with onset of symptoms at 11 to

17 years of age.[36,37] Only 1 toe is usually affected, with the second metatarsal being most commonly involved.[2,38]

Pathophysiology

Two major theories have been popularized as possible causes for Freiberg's disease, including trauma or vascular disruption. The original description by Freiberg in 1914 presented a traumatic basis for the etiology of the condition; this was later supported by Smillie and colleagues,[39] with note that patients with short first metatarsals, in a varus position or were hypermobile were at risk for the development of this condition.[40]

The second metatarsal receives its blood supply from the dorsal metatarsal artery and the medial deep plantar artery. Abnormalities in the vascular supply to the second metatarsal could predispose a patient to osteonecrosis of the metatarsal head in stressful environments.[36] Additionally, vascular compromise may result from mechanical compression, such as joint effusions, which could hinder blood flow in vessels perforating the joint capsule to reach the metatarsal head.[37]

Regardless of etiology, the end result is an ischemic epiphysis that initially fissures. Cancellous bone in the metatarsal head is resorbed leading to subchondral bone collapse. As central subchondral bone collapses, bony projections are left on either side. It is important to remember that the plantar-based cartilage remains intact. Ultimately, severe flattening of the head occurs with marked arthrosis of the metatarsophalangeal (MTP) joint.[39]

Clinical Findings

Patients often complain of pain in the region of the affected metatarsal head. They may report the sensation of walking on something akin to a pebble. The symptoms are often increased with barefoot walking. The toe may be swollen or elevated on physical examination; sagittal or coronal malalignment is not uncommon. Crepitus may be identified with passive range of motion of the MTP. Instability may be identified with Lachman testing of the affected joint.[36]

Imaging

Weight-bearing plain radiographs of the foot may demonstrate joint space widening early in the disease process. This may occur between 3 and 6 weeks after symptoms develop (**Fig. 9**).[41] With progression of the disease, metatarsal head flattening, central joint depression, and subchondral sclerosis may be seen (**Fig. 10**).[39] MRI can be a useful adjunct to evaluate for Freiberg's disease, when no changes are seen on plain films. Bone scan may also be used to identify regions of avascular bone.[36]

Treatment

Initial management is conservative, with a focus on symptom relief and minimizing stress to the injured metatarsal head. Modification of activities, antiinflammatories, and protected weight bearing can be used. Orthoses with metatarsal bars can offload the affected metatarsal head.[36] Cases refractory to nonoperative management may warrant operative intervention. The broad categories of surgical procedures are those that aim to alter the biomechanics or physiology (core decompression, osteotomies) or those procedures that aim to restore congruity to the joint to allay arthritic symptomatology (debridement, osteotomy, grafting, arthroplasty). Various degrees of efficacy have been reported with these procedures.

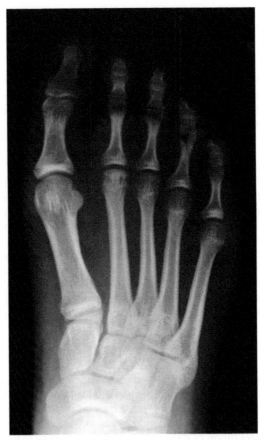

Fig. 9. Anteroposterior radiograph of the foot demonstrating early Freiberg's of the second metatarsal head.

Outcomes

For patients who are in the early stages of disease, conservative measures can be instituted with good response.[42] Surgical intervention can be used in refractory cases. Several reports exist documenting the utility of procedures available for treatment of Freiberg's disease. Core decompression aims to stimulate a vascular response and its use has been resulted in pain relief based on case reports in the literature.[43,44] Joint debridement with loose body removal has been found to have good results.[39,42,45] This can be completed via open or arthroscopic methods with comparable results.[46] Patients with earlier stages of the disease may be suitable for bone grafting, via a dorsal metatarsal shaft open-hinge technique. This has been reported to have good outcomes.[42] Osteotomies can be used to offload the metatarsal head (shortening) or to realign the joint (dorsiflexion). Smith and colleagues[47] used a shortening osteotomy to offload the metatarsal head and found 15 pf 16 patients experiences pain relief within 1 year of follow-up. Capar and colleagues[48] followed 19 patients for close to 4 years after completion of a dorsal closing wedge osteotomy. Although the technique is technically challenging and has the potential to produce a transfer lesion, the authors found good to excellent results in 84% of patients.[36] Arthroplasty procedures may involve either excision and/or interposition or a formal joint replacement.

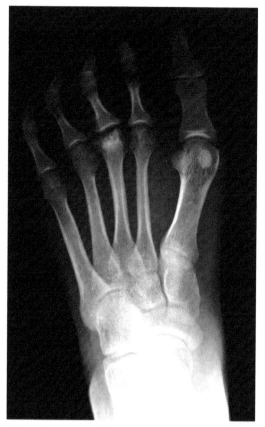

Fig. 10. Anteroposterior radiograph of the foot demonstrating late stage Freiberg's of the third metatarsal head.

Concerns with the excision include development of transfer metatarsalgia, MTP instability, hallux valgus, and shortening. Placement of interpositional grafts can help to maintain the joint space and avoid bony impingement during gait. Flexor tendons, extensor tendons, capsular tissue, and free grafts can be used.[36] Formal joint replacement has been reported with good results in 4 patients treated with a silicon implant.[49] Titanium has been used to develop a hemiarthroplasty implant and ceramic has been used to develop a total arthroplasty implant.[36,50] Possible complications include prosthetic failure, transfer lesions, silicon synovitis, osteolysis, infection, and sagittal malalignment.

COMPLEX REGIONAL PAIN SYNDROME
Epidemiology

Although the etiology of complex regional pain syndrome (CRPS) in children is not entirely clear, there have been recognized associations with chronic illness and psychological stressors.[51] CRPS was previously thought to be rare, likely secondary to under-recognition of the condition. In contrast with adults, the lower limb is much more frequently affected. The foot is the most commonly involved aspect of the lower extremity. Pediatric patients diagnosed with CRPS are often females who are in their late childhood to early adolescence.[52]

Pathophysiology

For most patients with CRPS, there is report of mild trauma. The exact events leading to the development of this pain syndrome are not completely understood.[52]

Clinical Findings

Patients may have difficulty bearing weight, evidence of allodynia, and autonomic system changes. The latter may manifest itself as excessive sweating, swelling, coolness to the skin, and mottling.

Imaging

Diagnostic studies are not often useful. Plain radiographs may show disuse osteopenic changes in chronic cases of disability. MRI may demonstrate localized marrow edema and bone scans may show limited signal uptake.[52]

Treatment

Management of CRPS is mostly symptomatic, including physical therapy for range of motion and strengthening of the affected extremity. More important, therapy helps to address desensitization against noxious stimuli.[51] This is often completed in conjunction with cognitive behavioral therapy to enable patients to improve coping skills with pain and other stressors.[52] For refractory cases, calcium channel blockers, antidepressants, or sympathetic nerve blocks may be useful.

Outcomes

Although the clinical literature is limited, there has been proven benefit to early mobilization and aggressive physical therapy. Sherry and colleagues[53] found a 92% resolution rate of initial symptoms in 103 patients using an intensive exercise program. Other studies have found that 70% of patients may require adjuvant medications (gabapentin or amitriptyline) to facilitate participation in physical therapy.[52]

SESAMOIDITIS
Epidemiology

Sesamoiditis is a challenging problem and can be a source of prolonged disability for the adolescent dancer. The medial sesamoid is most often involved.[54]

Pathophysiology

At the level of the MTP joint, 2 sesamoid bones are contained within the flexor hallucis brevis tendon. These bones articulate with the plantar aspect of the metatarsal head. The sesamoids experience substantial force as the dancer's foot moves through various positions, including, demi pointe, full pointe, and with jump landing. Excessive loading can occur with rolling in of the foot, pronation, and forced turn-out. Sesamoiditis often develops from repetitive injury.[55]

Clinical Findings

It is important to inquire about potential technical errors that may have taken place; there may be a reported history of an incorrect landing. On examination, there is pain with palpation of the medial sesamoid. Symptoms may be elicited when the examiner dorsiflexes the first MTP.[56] As the sesamoids move distally with great toe dorsiflexion, the pain may move distally as well.[54]

Imaging

Plain radiographs of the foot, including a sesamoid axial, are usually obtained. Acute fractures often have irregular edges and displacement of fracture fragments as opposed to a bipartite sesamoid, which has smoother cortical edges (**Fig. 11**). A bone scan can be obtained if radiographs are negative and clinical suspicion is high. CT can be used to evaluate sesamoid fracture nonunions and MRI can identify stress fractures.[57]

Treatment

Most patients respond well to nonoperative measures, including including a review of foot alignment/appropriate landing maneuvers and the use of antiinflammatories for pain control. Stiff-soled shoes can be used to limit motion of the MTP while a dancer is not in class.[54] Silicon pads can be affixed to the foot without affecting the use of ballet footwear. For refractory cases, operative intervention may be warranted.[57]

Outcomes

Resolution of pain with the sesamoids may take several months.[54]

OS TRIGONUM SYNDROME
Epidemiology

The accessory ossification center of the posterolateral talus (os trigonum) commonly appears in children between the ages of 8 and 11 years old. It typically fuses to the posterior talus within 1 year of its appearance. In 1 series that reported on 4 patients with pediatric os trigonum syndrome, 75% of the patients were female.[58] Affected patients are often involved with activities (ie, ballet, soccer) that required prolonged and forced plantarflexion of the ankle.[59]

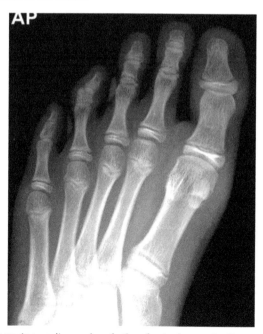

Fig. 11. Anteroposterior radiograph of the foot demonstrating a bipartite medial sesamoid.

Pathophysiology

Os trigonum may have a triangular, rounded, or oval type shape and is attached to the talus via fibers of the posterior talofibular ligament.[59] The persistence of the os trigonum has been attributed to a lack of fusion of the ossification center or a fracture nonunion.[60,61] Although the exact etiology of os trigonum syndrome is not clear, recurrent plantarflexion can lead to impingement of the os between the posterior tibia and calcaneus. This may drive the development of symptoms.[62]

Clinical Findings

Patients may note chronic pain either in the posterior ankle or in the foot for close to 1 year's duration.[59]

Imaging

Initial evaluation of the patient should begin with plain radiographs of the affected ankle (**Fig. 12**). Glard and colleagues[58] recommend obtaining a bone scan if the os trigonum is identified on the lateral radiograph of the ankle. A symptomatic os trigonum will have increased radiotracer uptake; MRI can be used subsequently to rule out other possible sources of chronic pain.[63] On MRI, edema within the os trigonum and increased diastasis between the os and the talus may be identified (**Fig. 13**). Other nonspecific findings on MRI include inflammation of the ankle joint posterior capsule and flexor hallucis longus tenosynovitis.[64]

Treatment

Although most os trigonums are asymptomatic, patients who develop symptoms should be initially treated with rest, activity modification, immobilization in a short leg cast or brace, and antiinflammatories.[59] If symptoms are refractory to conservative measures after a few weeks, surgical resection is considered. Surgical resection is most commonly performed via a posterolateral approach, which places the sural nerve at risk for injury. A posteromedial approach can be used, with appropriate concern for injury to the tibial neurovascular bundle.[58,65] Additionally, arthroscopic resection of the os trigonum can be performed.[66,67]

Outcomes

Although conservative measures may be useful, persistent symptoms for longer than 2 years may portend worse outcomes after surgical excision.[63] Subsequently surgical intervention should not be delayed when appropriate. Surgical excision using the posteromedial approach has been reported with clinical success and no incidence of neurovascular injury.[58,59] Use of arthroscopic techniques for excision of the

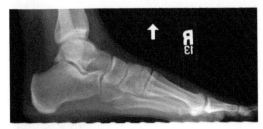

Fig. 12. Lateral radiograph of the foot demonstrating an os trigonum. The *arrow* indicates that the film is a weight bearing film. The *arrow* does not point to anything in particular just in the up direction.

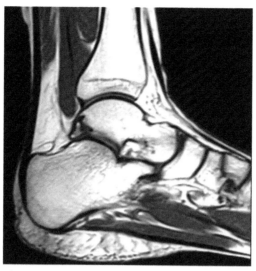

Fig. 13. Lateral MRI demonstrating an os trigonum.

symptomatic os trigonum has been associated with quicker recovery times, although the longer term results are comparable with open excision.[58,68]

FLEXIBLE FLATFOOT
Epidemiology

Flexible flat foot is typically a nonpainful condition that is commonly seen in children. The true incidence is not known.[69] Ninety percent of 1-year-old children seem to have flatfeet.[70] There is no evidence to suggest that the presence of flexible flatfeet will lead to the development of pain or arthritis.

Pathophysiology

The alignment and shape of the medial arch of the foot is determined by bony architecture and ligamentous laxity. The presence of a flexible flatfoot has been attributed to anatomic variations in composition of the medial arch of the foot. Most authors agree that the presence of excessive ligamentous laxity is part of the underlying mechanism for painless flexible flatfoot.[69]

Clinical Findings

Clinical evaluation of the patient with a painless flexible flatfoot should include a general musculoskeletal examination. This examination should include an evaluation of general ligamentous laxity of the patient. In most cases, this entity is painless; if there is pain, other causes should be investigated. There is often valgus of the hindfoot, supination of the forefoot, and a tight Achilles tendon. The medial longitudinal arch will reconstitute when the patient is asked to stand on their tiptoes, as a result of contraction of the posterior tibial tendon and activation of the windlass mechanism via the plantar fascia.[69]

Imaging

Standard weight-bearing radiographs of the foot can help to guide diagnosis but are not essential; this includes standing anteroposterior, lateral, and oblique views. On an anteroposterior radiograph, the talocalcaneal angle (along the longitudinal axes of each bone) will be greater than 55°. On a lateral view the talocalcaneal angle (along the longitudinal axis of each bone) will also be greater than 55°. The most commonly used angle to quantify sag of the medial column is the Meary's angle. This angle, which is evaluated on a lateral radiograph of the foot, represents the angle between the talus and first metatarsal. This angle is typically 0°; however, no standards for normal angles are accepted in the pediatric population. Most important, the magnitude of the angles neither correlates with symptoms or the need for treatment.[71]

Treatment

The mainstay of treatment of the painless flexible flatfoot is observation, reassurance, and education. Additionally, heel cord stretching should be utilized to help address contracture of the Achilles and its contribution to hindfoot valgus.[69]

Although a variety of corrective/symptomatic orthoses (sneakers, heel cups, shoe inserts, custom molded plastics inserts, etc) can be used, there has been no evidence indicating that their use has any impact on painless flexible flatfoot outcomes.[72] In the uncommon case of a progressively painful flat foot with a tight heel cord that not does respond to conservative treatment, surgery may be indicated. The most common surgical procedure includes a calcaneal lengthening osteotomy and an Achilles tendon lengthening.[69]

Outcomes

Multiple studies have demonstrated that treatment of painless flexible flatfoot has no influence on outcome.[73,74] Wenger and colleagues[72] followed children for approximately 5 years and could not find any effect of shoe modifications compared with matched controls. No literature is presently available to ascertain the impact of the Achilles stretching on the natural history of painless flexible flat foot.

REFERENCES

1. DiGiovanni CW, Patel A, Calfee R, et al. Osteonecrosis in the foot. J Am Acad Orthop Surg 2007;15(4):208–17.
2. Gillespie H. Osteochondroses and apophyseal injuries of the foot in the young athlete. Curr Sports Med Rep 2010;9(5):265–8.
3. Ippolito E, Ricciardi Pollini PT, Falez F. Koehler's disease of the tarsal navicular: long-term follow-up of 12 cases. J Pediatr Orthop 1984;4:416–7.
4. Williams GA, Cowell HR. Kohler's disease of the tarsal navicular. Clin Orthop Relat Res 1981;158:53–8.
5. Cahill BR. Chronic orthopaedic problems in the young athlete. J Sports Med 1973;1:36–9.
6. Ogden JA, Ganey TM, Hill JD, et al. Sever's injury: a stress fracture of the immature calcaneal metaphysis. J Pediatr Orthop 2004;24:488–92.
7. Micheli LJ, Ireland ML. Prevention and management of calcaneal apophysitis in children: an overuse syndrome. J Pediatr Orthop 1987;7(1):34–8.
8. Wiegerinck JI, Yntema C, Brouwer HJ, et al. Incidence of calcaneal apophysitis in the general population. Eur J Pediatr 2014;173(5):677–9.
9. Pommering TL, Kluchurosky L, Hall SL. Ankle and foot injuries in pediatric and adult athletes. Prim Care 2005;32:133–61.
10. Staheli LT. Footwear for children. Instr Course Lect 1994;43:193–7.
11. Canale ST, Williams KD. Iselin's disease. J Pediatr Orthop 1992;12(1):90–3.
12. Lehman RC, Gregg JR, Torg E. Iselin's disease. Am J Sports Med 1986;14:494–6.

13. Stormont DM, Peterson HA. The relative incidence of tarsal coalition. Clin Orthop Relat Res 1983;181:28–36.
14. Mubarak SJ, Patel PN, Upasani VV, et al. Calcaneonavicular coalition: treatment by excision and fat graft. J Pediatr Orthop 2009;29(5):418–26.
15. Zaw H, Calder JD. Tarsal coalitions. Foot Ankle Clin 2010;15:349–64.
16. Plotkin S. Case presentation of calcaneonavicular coalition in monozygotic twins. J Am Podiatr Med Assoc 1996;86(9):433–8.
17. Conway JJ, Cowell HR. Tarsal coalition: clinical significance and roentgenographic demonstration. Radiology 1969;92:799–811.
18. Cowell HR. Tarsal coalition—review and update. Instr Course Lect 1982;31: 264–71.
19. Mosier KM, Asher M. Tarsal coalitions and peroneal spastic flatfoot: a review. J Bone Joint Surg Am 1984;66:976–84.
20. Swiontkowski MF, Scranton PE, Hansen S. Tarsal coalitions: long-term results of surgical treatment. J Pediatr Orthop 1983;3:287–92.
21. Lemley F, Berlet G, Hill K, et al. Current concepts review: tarsal coalition. Foot Ankle Int 2006;27(12):1163–9.
22. Mann RA, Baumgarten M. Subtalar fusion for isolated subtalar disorders: preliminary report. Clin Orthop 1988;226:260–5.
23. Varner KE, Michelson JD. Tarsal coalition in adults. Foot Ankle Int 2000;21: 669–72.
24. Comfort TK, Johnson LO. Resection for symptomatic talocalcaneal coalition. J Pediatr Orthop 1998;18(3):283–8.
25. Wilde PH, Torode IP, Dickens DR, et al. Resection for symptomatic talocalcaneal coalition. J Bone Joint Surg Br 1994;76(5):797–801.
26. Leonard ZC, Fortin PT. Adolescent accessory navicular. Foot Ankle Clin 2010; 15:337–47.
27. Coskun N, Yuksel M, Cevener M, et al. Incidence of accessory ossicles and sesamoid bones in the feet: a radiographical study of the Turkish subjects. Surg Radiol Anat 2009;31(1):19–24.
28. Coughlin MJ. Sesamoids and accessory bones of the foot. In: Coughlin MJ, Mann RA, Saltzman CL, editors. Surgery of the foot and ankle. 8th edition. Philadelphia: Mosby; 2007. p. 531–610.
29. Mygind H. The accessory tarsal scaphoid; clinical features and treatment. Acta Orthop Scand 1953;23(2):142–51.
30. Sullivan JA, Miller WA. The relationship of the accessory navicular to the development of the flat foot. Clin Orthop 1979;144:233–7.
31. Veitch JM. Evaluation of the Kidner procedure in treatment of symptomatic accessory tarsal scaphoid. Clin Orthop 1978;131:210–3.
32. Macnicol MF, Voutsinas S. Surgical treatment of the symptomatic accessory navicular. J Bone Joint Surg Br 1984;66:218–26.
33. Nakayama S, Sugimoto K, Takakura Y, et al. Percutaneous drilling of symptomatic accessory navicular in young athletes. Am J Sports Med 2005;33:531–5.
34. Scott AT, Sabesan VJ, Saluta JR, et al. Fusion versus excision of the symptomatic type II accessory navicular: a prospective study. Foot Ankle Int 2009;30: 10–5.
35. Chung JW, Chu IT. Outcome of fusion of a painful accessory navicular to the primary navicular. Foot Ankle Int 2009;30(2):106–9.
36. Cerrato RA. Freiberg's disease. Foot Ankle Clin 2011;16(4):647–58.
37. Carmont MR, Rees RJ, Blundell CM. Current concepts review: Freiberg's disease. Foot Ankle Int 2009;30:167–76.

38. Gauthier G, Elbaz R. Freiberg's infraction: a subchondral bone fatigue fracture. A new surgical treatment. Clin Orthop Relat Res 1979;93:93–5.

39. Smillie IS. Treatment of Freiberg's infraction. Proc R Soc Med 1967;60:29–31.

40. Freiberg AH. Infraction of the second metatarsal bone, a typical injury. Surg Gynecol Obstet 1914;19:191–3.

41. Hill J, Jimenez LA, Langford JH. Osteochondritis dissecans treated by joint replacement. J Am Podiatry Assoc 1979;69:556–61.

42. Helal B, Gibb P. Freiberg's disease: a suggested pattern of management. Foot Ankle Int 1987;8:94–102.

43. Dolce M, Osher L, McEneaney P, et al. The use of surgical core decompression as treatment for avascular necrosis of the second and third metatarsal heads. Foot 2006;17:162–6.

44. Fieberg AA, Fieberg RA. Core decompression as a novel approach treatment for early Freiberg's infraction of the second metatarsal head. Orthopedics 1995;18:1177–8.

45. Freiberg AH. The so-called infraction of the second metatarsal bone. J Bone Joint Surg Br 1926;8:257–61.

46. Carro LP, Golano P, Farinas O, et al. Arthroscopic Keller technique for Freiberg disease. Arthroscopy 2004;20:60–3.

47. Smith TWD, Stanley D, Rowley DI. Treatment of Freiberg's disease: a new operative technique. J Bone Joint Surg Br 1991;73:129–30.

48. Capar B, Kutluay E, Mujde S. Dorsal closing-wedge osteotomy in the treatment of Freiberg's disease. Acta Orthop Traumatol Turc 2007;41:136–9.

49. Cracchiolo A, Kitaoka HB, Leventen EO. Silicone implant arthroplasty for second metatarsophalangeal joint disorders with and without hallux valgus. Foot Ankle Int 1988;9:10–8.

50. Townshend DN, Greiss ME. Total ceramic arthroplasty for painful destructive disorders of the lesser metatarso-phalangeal joints. Foot 2006;17:73.

51. Houghton KM. Review for the generalist: evaluation of pediatric foot and ankle pain. Pediatr Rheumatol Online J 2008;6:6.

52. Low AK, Ward K, Wines AP. Pediatric complex regional pain syndrome. J Pediatr Orthop 2007;27(5):567–72.

53. Sherry D. Short and long-term outcomes of children with complex regional pain syndrome type 1 treated with exercise therapy. Clin J Pain 1999;15:218–23.

54. Kadel NJ. Foot and ankle injuries in dance. Phys Med Rehabil Clin N Am 2006; 17(4):813–26.

55. Macintyre J, Joy E. Foot and ankle injuries in dance. Clin Sports Med 2000; 19(2):351–68.

56. Van Hal ME, Keene JS, Lange TA, et al. Stress fractures of the great toe sesamoids. Am J Sports Med 1982;10(2):122–8.

57. Brown TD, Micheli LJ. Foot and ankle injuries in dance. Am J Orthop (Belle Mead NJ) 2004;33(6):303–9.

58. Glard Y, Jacopin S, de Landevoisin ES, et al. Symptomatic os trigonum in children. Foot Ankle Surg 2009;15(2):82–5.

59. de Landevoisin ES, Jacopin S, Glard Y, et al. Surgical treatment of the symptomatic os trigonum in children. Orthop Traumatol Surg Res 2009;95(2):159–63.

60. Shepherd FJ. A hitherto undescribed fracture of the astragalus. J Anat Physiol 1882;17:79–81.

61. Turner W. A secondary astragalus in the human foot. J Anat Physiol 1882;17:82–3.

62. Horibe S, Kita K, Natsu-ume T, et al. A novel technique of arthroscopic excision of a symptomatic os trigonum. Arthroscopy 2008;24(121):e121–4.

63. Abramowitz Y, Wollstein RY, London E, et al. Outcome of resection of a symptomatic os trigonum. J Bone Joint Surg Am 2003;85-A:1051–7.
64. Tamburrini O, Porpiglia H, Barresi D, et al. The role of magnetic resonance in the diagnosis of the os trigonum syndrome. Radiol Med 1999;98:462–7.
65. Brodsky AE, Khalil MA. Talar compression syndrome. Am J Sports Med 1986;14: 472–6.
66. Lombardi CM, Silhanek AD, Connolly FG. Modified arthroscopic excision of the symptomatic os trigonum and release of the flexor hallucis longus tendon: operative technique and case study. J Foot Ankle Surg 1999;38:347–51.
67. Marumoto JM, Ferkel RD. Arthroscopicexcisionoftheostrigonum:a new technique with preliminary clinical results. Foot Ankle Int 1997;18:777–84.
68. Jerosch J, Fadel M. Endoscopic resection of a symptomatic os trigonum. Knee Surg Sports Traumatol Arthrosc 2006;14:1188–93.
69. Mosca VS. Flexible flatfoot in children and adolescents. J Child Orthop 2010;4: 107–21.
70. Morley AJ. Knock-knee in children. Br Med J 1957;2:976–9.
71. Vanderwilde R, Staheli LT, Chew DE, et al. Measurements on radiographs of the foot in normal infants and children. J Bone Joint Surg Am 1988;70:407–15.
72. Wenger DR, Mauldin D, Speck G, et al. Corrective shoes and inserts as treatment for flexible flatfoot in infants and children. J Bone Joint Surg Am 1989; 71:800–10.
73. Gould N, Moreland M, Alvarez R, et al. Development of the child's arch. Foot Ankle 1989;9:241–5.
74. Sim-Fook L, Hodgson AR. A comparison of foot forms among the non-shoe and shoe-wearing Chinese population. J Bone Joint Surg Am 1958;40:1058–62.

Evaluation and Treatment of Childhood Musculoskeletal Injury in the Office

Peter J. Apel, MD, PhD[a],*, Andrew Howard, MD, MSc, FRCSC[b],*

KEYWORDS

- Office • Treatment • Musculoskeletal injury • Children

KEY POINTS

- History and examination should be focused.
- Radiographs should be obtained if the diagnosis is in question.
- Most pediatric injuries can be treated with office-based modalities.
- It is important for primary care providers to be able to distinguish the common stable injuries from those that require urgent orthopedic referral.

INTRODUCTION

Evaluation and treatment of acute musculoskeletal injuries can be rewarding for primary care providers. They are common presenting complaints and, with appropriate management, many patients make a full recovery in a short period of time. This article reviews basic principles of evaluation of acutely injured children, treatment strategies, and common injuries, and gives an overview of similar but more dangerous conditions that require referral.

LOCATION OF EVALUATION: OFFICE OR HOSPITAL?

Many pediatric musculoskeletal injuries are the result of ground-level falls, recreational sports, and other low-energy mechanisms. Most of these injuries can be treated nonoperatively with readily available supplies, especially in young children in whom skeletal growth is still occurring.

In general, low-energy injuries can usually be managed an office setting, whereas moderate-energy or high-energy injuries are more appropriate for hospital-based

[a] Orthopaedics, Guthrie, 130 Center Way, Corning, NY 14830, USA; [b] Division of Orthopedic Surgery, Hospital for Sick Children, 555 University Avenue, Toronto, Ontario M5G1X8, Canada
* Corresponding authors.
E-mail addresses: dr.peter.apel@gmail.com; andrew.howard@sickkids.ca

Pediatr Clin N Am 61 (2014) 1207–1222
http://dx.doi.org/10.1016/j.pcl.2014.08.009
0031-3955/14/$ – see front matter © 2014 Elsevier Inc. All rights reserved.

pediatric.theclinics.com

evaluation and management. Factors that increase the energy associated with an injury include increasing age, weight, and size of the child. Falls from heights, bicycles, trampolines, and bunk beds are often moderate-energy injuries and occasionally require advanced care. Injuries from motorized vehicles (motorcycle, car, all-terrain vehicle, snowmobile) should be evaluated in a hospital setting.

HISTORY

For children presenting with acute injuries, the history should be focused and not overly broad. The limited history should contain the mechanism of injury, location of pain, and any associated injuries. Injuries occasionally are associated with a pop, snap, or deformity. Details regarding the position of the limb at the time of maximal injury or displacement can reveal the energy imparted during injury. An important aspect of the history is the ability to bear weight after the injury. Inability to bear weight is often an indicator of severe injury, and should have a lower threshold for referral. Patients often do not try to bear weight after the injury. If radiographs are negative for fracture, patients should be encouraged to attempt weight bearing after a short period (2–3 days) of rest. Fractures may be evident as bent or crumpled bones; **Box 1** and **Fig. 1** give examples of plastic deformation.

PHYSICAL EXAMINATION

Much like the history, the physical examination should be focused on the area of injury and not be overly broad. Inspection and palpation are often all that is needed to make an accurate diagnosis.

Begin with inspection for deformity, swelling, and ecchymosis. In order to gain trust with injured children, first ask them to show where they hurt and to show their active range of motion. Carefully palpate for tenderness above and below the point of maximum tenderness. If the patient tolerates it, passive range of motion can be assessed.

As with all injuries, a focused and vascular examination should be performed. Function of the major nerves of the extremities as well as palpation for pulses should be performed. Any neurologic or vascular deficit should immediately be referred to the emergency department for evaluation.

Provocative maneuvers should not be performed in acutely injured patients, because these maneuvers are often painful and can be falsely negative, which is misleading in an acute swollen joint. These maneuvers include the Lachman test, anterior and posterior drawer tests, and stressing of injured joints. If major ligamentous injury is suspected, the patient should receive initial treatment and reexamination in a delayed manner.

RADIOGRAPHS

Radiograph examination of the injured anatomic area is an important aspect of acute injury evaluation. With modern radiographic techniques, the radiation dose is minimal, and every consideration ought to be given to obtaining appropriate radiographs of the affected area. Radiographic diagnosis is often straightforward and there are many clinically indistinguishable injuries that are easily discernible with proper radiographs (eg, a pelvic apophyseal avulsion from a slipped capital femoral epiphysis [SCFE]). Whenever the pelvis or hips are being examined radiographically, bilateral views, including frog laterals, are necessary.

However, some common injuries do not necessitate radiographs either at initial evaluation or at follow-up. Low-risk ankle injuries (which are usually simple sprains) do not require radiographs. A low-risk ankle injury includes an injury with tenderness

---

Box 1
Examination, treatments, and injury types

History and physical examination
- The history and physical examination should be focused and not overly broad
- Inability to bear weight may indicate a severe injury
- The point of maximum tenderness should be identified
- Joints proximal and distal to the point of maximum tenderness should be palpated

Office-based treatments
- Stable injuries can be treated with readily available medical supplies
- Slings, removable splints, rigid plastic boots, tape, and crutches
- Treatment is symptom directed and can be discontinued when symptoms subside

Knee injuries
- Key: ability to bear weight
- Radiographs are not always needed
- Minor injuries can be treated with rest, ice, and observation
- Severe injuries should be referred to an orthopedic surgeon

Ankle injuries
- Key: ability to bear weight
- Radiographs are not always needed
- Minor injuries can be treated with removable walking boots

Proximal humerus and clavicle fractures
- Most are treated in a simple sling with return to activities as tolerated
- Adolescents with displaced or angulated fractures should be referred

Elbow fractures
- Low threshold for referral to a pediatric orthopedic surgeon
- Proper radiographs, with careful inspection of the radiographs to avoid missing injuries

Hand fractures
- Metacarpal fractures should be referred
- Finger fractures can often be treated with buddy taping
- Thumb fractures can often be treated in removable thumb spica splints

---

and swelling isolated to the distal fibula and/or the ligaments immediately adjacent to the fibula. In these cases, an ankle radiograph is unnecessary, and the clinical diagnosis of ankle sprain can be made.[1] Acute knee injuries wherein the patient can bear weight similarly do not necessitate radiographs.[2] After initial radiographic diagnosis, buckle fractures and most foot, toe, and finger fractures do not need radiographs at follow-up if there is no clinical deformity.

PLASTIC DEFORMITY

Pediatric bone is physiologically different from adult bone because of a myriad of biochemical and histologic factors. Injury often involves plastic deformation of the

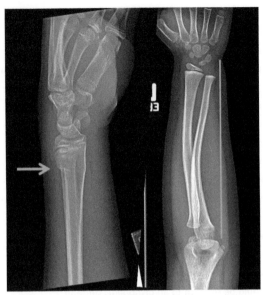

Fig. 1. Plastic deformation. Soft pediatric bone may simply undergo deformation rather than complete fracturing. On the left is a typical distal radius fracture (*arrow*) with the dorsal cortex deformed and buckled giving this fracture its name. On the right is an injury to the forearm that has deformed the ulna (which is usually straight).

bone with or without adjacent fracture. Most of these plastic deformations and fractures are stable and require no specific intervention, but it is important to understand the full injury and not miss an associated dislocation. A common location for plastic deformation is the forearm. In some cases, the ulna may be deformed and the radial head dislocated (Monteggia variant).

OFFICE-BASED TREATMENTS

Many minor injuries in children can be treated with readily available off-the-shelf medical equipment including slings, removable splints, tape (for finger and toe fractures), crutches, and off-the-shelf rigid walking boots. A small supply of these items can be stocked in the office, or patients can be referred to local pharmacies and instructed in their use.

Slings

Simple slings are a common treatment of upper extremity injuries. They are the preferred treatment of most shoulder, proximal humerus, and clavicle fractures. A simple sling is equivalent to more sophisticated alternatives in clavicle fractures.[3] Slings should be used judiciously in young children, because often they are an encumbrance rather than an aid. In adolescents, slings are less problematic. Slings are for comfort and may be discontinued when symptoms subside.

Removable Splints

Removable splints are commercially available in a wide range of sizes and are an appropriate treatment of wrist (**Fig. 2**), thumb, finger, and toe fractures. The general goal of the removable splint is to provide a moderate amount of comfort and

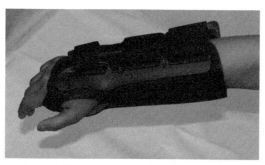

Fig. 2. Removable wrist splint. The removable wrist splint is widely available, and is appropriate for most injuries about the wrist. Removable thumb spica splint are also available and can be used to treat hand fractures, including stable thumb metacarpal or phalangeal.

immobilization while allowing easy bathing and hygiene. These splints provide support and reassurance and are generally best for stable fractures. Removable splints can generally be discontinued when symptoms subside.

Rigid Plastic Boot

The rigid plastic boot (**Fig. 3**) is the mainstay product for treatment of stable lower extremity injuries. Boots come in a wide range of sizes, shapes, and names. The following names all refer to a rigid plastic boot: fracture boot, cam walker, high-tide

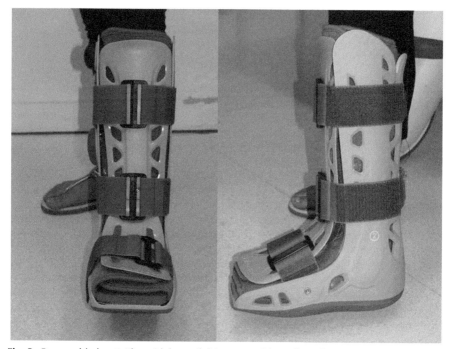

Fig. 3. Removable boot. The widely available removable walking boot comes in a variety of sizes and shapes and from numerous vendors. It is an excellent treatment of stable injuries below the knee.

boot, low-tide boot, and so forth. Regardless of the manufacturer or nomenclature, the general purpose is to immobilize the ankle and foot. It is a type of removable splint, and again is best for stable injuries. The removable nature of the boot allows for bathing, hygiene, and like other removable splints its use can be discontinued when symptoms subside.

Buddy Taping

Buddy taping is standard of care for stable finger and toe phalangeal fractures. The basic principle is that the intact neighboring digit serves as a splint for the injured digit. Small strips of tape are applied between the joints of the two digits to be taped together. Two strips of tape between the adjacent proximal and middle phalanges are usually sufficient to immobilize the digit. Patients are encouraged to then use the buddy-taped fingers together as a unit. Taping can be discontinued when symptoms subside.

Crutches

Crutches are an appropriate treatment whenever lower extremity weight bearing should be limited, either because of pain or following medical instruction. Crutches are widely available at medical supply stores and pharmacies. Although most adolescents have the gross motor skills to use crutches effectively, smaller children often need some instruction. Simple in-office nursing education on the use of crutches is usually sufficient. Patients who are new to crutches should be shown how to go up and down stairs safely and show basic proficiency. For most stable injuries, patients should be encouraged to start by using both crutches to stay completely off the painful extremity, and then graduate to using 1 crutch (on the opposite side to the affected limb). As symptoms allow, patients can progress weight bearing until crutches are no longer needed.

LOWER EXTREMITY
Pelvis, Hip, and Femur

Injuries to the pelvis, hip, and femur are uncommon in the primary care provider's office. Major injuries are debilitating and painful and are usually seen in the emergency department setting. Two injuries that can be seen in the primary care office are apophyseal avulsion fractures and SCFE. Both are more common in adolescents. The clinical diagnosis of a groin pull in any adolescent patient should be proved radiographically not to be an SCFE before proceeding with treatment.

Apophyseal Avulsion Fractures

Apophyseal avulsion fractures are common in adolescents, especially in athletes, and are often associated with an acute event such as twisting or a fall. Patients often hear a pop about the hip. These injuries are painful and patients often refuse to bear weight. Radiograph findings are convincing. Common locations for apophyseal avulsions include the anterior superior iliac spine (ASIS) (**Fig. 4**), anterior inferior iliac spine, iliac crest, and the ischial tuberosity. Treatment is generally supportive: crutches as needed for 4 to 6 weeks, limited activity, and ice. These injuries do not require orthopedic referral. Patients can be told that symptoms will begin to subside within 2 weeks, with most symptoms usually resolved by 8 to 10 weeks. If symptoms persist beyond 12 weeks, orthopedic referral should be considered.

Slipped Capital Femoral Epiphysis

Any adolescent who presents with pain around the groin, femur, or even to the knee should be evaluated for an SCFE. These injuries are well known for vague pain,

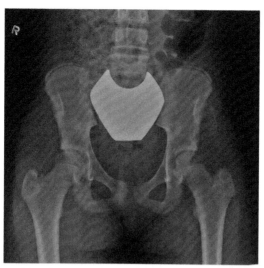

Fig. 4. Apophyseal avulsion fracture. Note the left-sided avulsion of the ASIS.

radiating pain, and for masquerading as groin pulls. Failure to diagnose appropriately can lead to serious consequences if severe acute slippage occurs. This diagnosis is best made on lateral radiographs, so radiographs should always be ordered as an anteroposterior pelvis with a bilateral frog lateral. **Fig. 5** shows an example of radiographic findings of SCFE. Patients found to have an SCFE should immediately be instructed to be non–weight bearing with crutches and need urgent orthopedic referral or to be sent to the emergency department.

KNEE
Acute Knee Injury

Acute knee injuries are common after sports injuries. These injuries should be triaged based on severity. If patients can bear weight, radiographs are not necessary.[2]

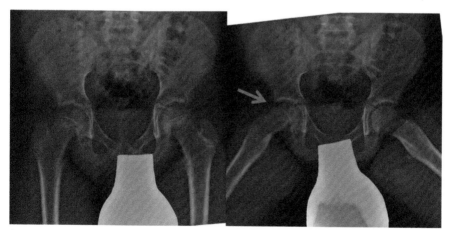

Fig. 5. SCFE. Note the right-sided SCFE (*arrow*) which is best seen in the frog lateral view, and that there is a clear difference from the contralateral side.

If patients can bear weight, or if they cannot bear weight but radiographs are negative, a period of watchful observation is appropriate. These minor knee injuries can be treated with rest, ice, range of motion as tolerated, and gradual turn to sport. Most acute sprains resolve within 2 to 3 weeks. If symptoms do not resolve, magnetic resonance imaging (MRI) should be considered and referral to orthopedic surgeon should be made. MRI findings of a complete anterior cruciate ligament rupture are shown in **Fig. 6**.

Acute knee injuries associated with large effusion, inability to bear weight, limitations in range of motion, or mechanical symptoms such as catching or locking and popping should receive preliminary evaluation and temporizing treatment with a knee immobilizer and crutches. Referral to orthopedic surgeon is appropriate for these more severe injuries.

Fractures About the Knee and Tibial Shaft

Fractures about the knee usually require orthopedic referral, because these are often treated operatively or in fiberglass casts. These injuries include distal femur buckle fractures, proximal tibial buckle fractures, tibial spine avulsion fractures, patellar fractures, tibial tubercle avulsion fractures, and tibial shaft fractures, including the toddler's fracture. These fractures should be referred to a pediatric orthopedic surgeon for evaluation and management. **Fig. 7** shows radiographic findings of tibial spine and tibial tubercle avulsion fractures, which occur only in children. **Fig. 8** shows pediatric patterns of tibial shaft fractures, including a toddler's fracture and a buckle fracture.

Ankle Injuries

Ankle injuries are common to all ages, and vary in severity. Fractures involving the ankle mortise or closing distal tibia physis are common in adolescents, and should be evaluated and managed by a pediatric orthopedic surgeon. In general, inability to bear weight is an indicator of a more severe injury. For more minor injuries with which the patient can bear weight and has no bony tenderness, radiographs are not always necessary,[1] and treatments can be symptom directed.

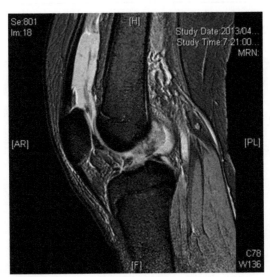

Fig. 6. Acute knee injury (severe). MRI shows a large effusion and a complete tear of the anterior cruciate ligament.

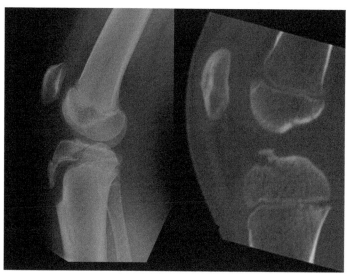

Fig. 7. Knee fractures. (*Left*) Proximal tibial tubercle fracture. (*Right*) Tibial spine avulsion fracture.

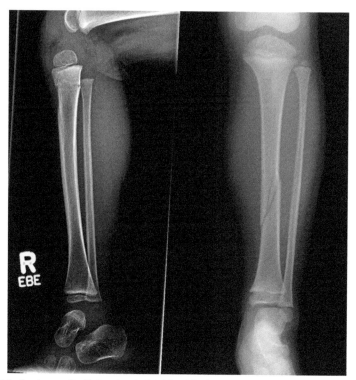

Fig. 8. Tibia fractures. (*Left*) Proximal tibial buckle fracture. (*Right*) Toddler's fracture.

In the past, it was thought that isolated lateral ankle injuries with negative radiographs represented a nondisplaced Salter-Harris I physeal injury of the distal fibula. However, a recent study showed this to be extremely unusual[1]; far more common is the routine ankle sprain or contusion.[4] These injuries can be treated in a removable boot with weight bearing as tolerated, range of motion, and return to activities as symptoms allow. Persistent pain or failure to make a quick recovery should prompt a referral to an orthopedic surgeon.

Foot and Toes

Foot injuries can be caused by a variety mechanisms, and include metatarsal fractures and phalangeal fractures. Most metatarsal fractures can be treated in a removable boot. Toe fractures of the proximal or middle phalanges are pretreated with buddy taping, weight bearing as tolerated, and return to activities when symptoms resolve. **Fig. 9** shows metatarsal and phalangeal fractures in the foot.

Seymour fracture

A unique fracture that can be seen in skeletally immature toes is the Seymour fracture. First described in the distal phalanges of the hand, this is an injury that involves the physis of the distal phalanx and the overlying nail bed. This injury may present as a severe stubbed toe with bleeding from the base of the nail bed. It is an open fracture and the overlying nail bed is often incarcerated within the growth plate of the distal phalanx. It is important to recognize this injury, because it requires urgent referral, open irrigation debridement, and fixation. Failure to identify and treat this can lead to deep infection. For the primary care provider, the key points regarding this injury are early recognition and prompt referral.

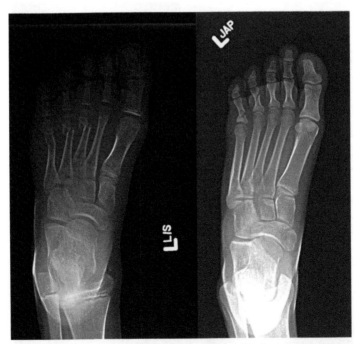

Fig. 9. Foot fractures. (*Left*) Three metatarsal fractures, effectively treated in a removable boot. (*Right*) Proximal phalanx fractures of the fourth and fifth digit, treated with buddy taping.

UPPER EXTREMITY
Shoulder

Clavicle fractures

Most acute injuries to the shoulder are caused by a fall on an outstretched extremity. The most common injuries include clavicle fractures and proximal humerus fractures. Unlike adults, children do not usually get acromioclavicular (AC) joint sprains or rotator cuff injuries. The AC joint sprain equivalent in a growing child is a separation of the distal clavicle epiphysis. This injury heals via the intact periosteum and forms a neoclavicle, as shown in **Fig. 10**. Most clavicle fractures in children can be treated nonoperatively, but there is controversy regarding treatment of clavicle fractures in adolescents.[5] If nonoperative treatment is chosen, a simple sling is sufficient. The historically used figure-of-eight bandage is unnecessary.[3] A sling is used for comfort until pain has subsided enough that range of motion can be tolerated. Patients can start with gentle pendulum exercises and progress range of motion and activities as tolerated. Eight to 12 weeks is usually sufficient healing time to return to sports.

Proximal humerus fractures

Similar to clavicle fractures, most proximal humerus fractures are treated nonoperatively. In young children, these can be treated with a simple sling, with the gradual weaning out of the sling and range of motion as tolerated. In adolescents with little growth remaining and significant displacement, referral to an orthopedic surgeon should be made. For nonoperative treatment, a simple sling should be used for comfort for 1 to 2 weeks, with increasing range of motion as tolerated, and a return to full activities within 8 to 12 weeks. **Fig. 11** shows examples of proximal humerus fractures at different ages.

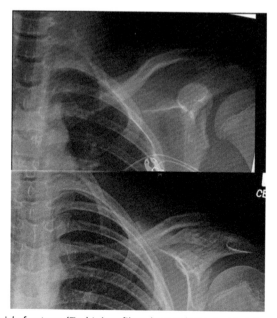

Fig. 10. Distal clavicle fracture. (*Top*) Injury films show a distal clavicle injury, mimicking an AC joint separation. (*Bottom*) Four weeks later, the periosteal sleeve has formed a neoclavicle.

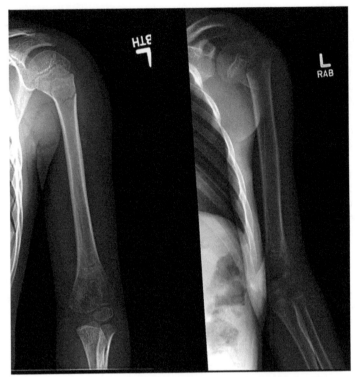

Fig. 11. Proximal humerus fractures. (*Left*) A minimally displaced proximal humerus fracture in a 4-year-old child. This injury is appropriate for a simple sling. (*Right*) A displaced and angulated proximal humerus fracture in a 14-year-old. This injury should be referred to an orthopedic surgeon for management.

Elbow

The elbow is a common area of injury in children, and one of particular consternation for emergency physicians, radiologists, and pediatricians because of concern regarding missing an injury that requires surgery. For this reason, most elbow fractures in children should be referred to a pediatric orthopedic surgeon for management. These injuries include supracondylar humerus fractures, lateral condyle fractures, radial neck fractures, and olecranon fractures. For a nondisplaced supracondylar humerus fracture, the telltale anterior and posterior fat pad signs are often the only findings on radiographs, as shown in **Fig. 12**.

For the primary care provider, there are 2 elbow injuries of particular note, because they are often missed: (1) Monteggia injury, and (2) the lateral condyle fracture. Both Monteggia injuries and lateral condyle fractures can be subtle, with mild to moderate amounts of pain and minimal bruising. There may still be range of motion of the elbow with these injuries. The pathognomonic finding for a Monteggia injury is dislocation of the radiocapitellar joint. This injury is best appreciated on a lateral radiograph, on which a line drawn on the shaft of the radius does not intersect the capitellum (**Fig. 13**). These injuries should be promptly referred to an orthopedic surgeon. In order to better identify lateral condyle fractures, full radiographs, including internal rotation oblique (**Fig. 14**), should be ordered.[6] Particular attention should be paid to the lateral radiograph, and any visible fracture, however small, should be referred to an orthopedic surgeon.

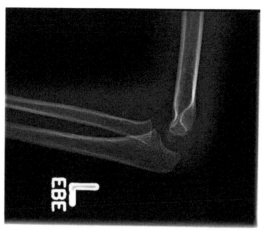

Fig. 12. Supracondylar humerus fracture. This lateral radiograph shows a nondisplaced supracondylar humerus fracture. Note the anterior and posterior fat pad signs.

Forearm

Similar to elbow injuries, most forearm fractures are referred to pediatric orthopedic surgeons for management. Exceptions include nondisplaced or buckle-type fractures of the distal third of the forearm that are minimally displaced. These injuries can be treated similarly to wrist buckle fractures, as discussed later. Any displacement or angulation in the shaft of the radius or ulna should be referred to a pediatric orthopedic surgeon for management.

Wrist

Buckle fractures

Perhaps the most common injury seen the pediatric office is the distal radius buckle fracture. This injury is often caused by falling on an outstretched hand. Lateral

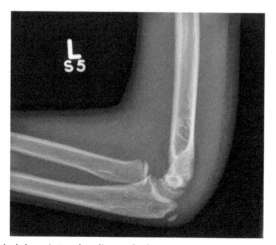

Fig. 13. Monteggia injury. Lateral radiograph shows a Monteggia injury that was initially missed. There were no bony fractures, but note that the radial head is anteriorly dislocated in relation to the capitellum.

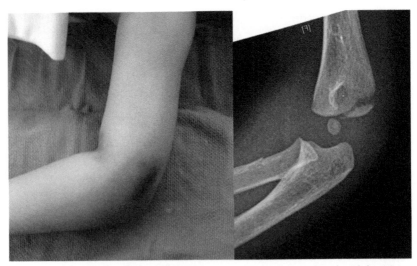

Fig. 14. Lateral condyle fracture. These injuries are commonly associated with bruising over the lateral elbow. The internal rotation radiograph shows displacement of the lateral condyle fracture. These injuries are usually managed operatively.

radiographs best show the fracture, as shown in **Fig. 15**. These fractures may have up to 15° to 20° of angulation. However, the angulation is in the metaphysis near the growth plate and usually, with subsequent skeletal growth, the angular deformity remodels.

Buckle fracture of the wrist is a stable injury, and requires little intervention other than rest, ice, reassurance, and a soft bandage or removable splint. Fractures with less than 15° to 20° of angulation do not require operative intervention, reduction under anesthetic, or orthopedic consultation. It has been shown in several level I

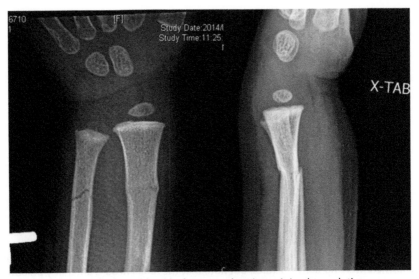

Fig. 15. Buckle fracture. Typical buckle fractures showing minimal angulation.

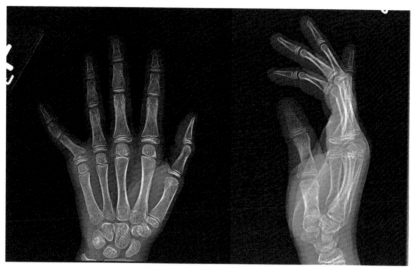

Fig. 16. Finger fractures. (*Left*) Minimally displaced Salter-Harris II fracture of the proximal phalanx of the little finger. This injury can be treated with buddy taping. (*Right*) Minimally displaced Salter-Harris II fracture of the proximal phalanx of the thumb. This injury can be treated with a removable thumb spica splint.

studies that hard casts are not better than a soft bandage or a removable splint.[7–9] These fractures should be managed in the primary care provider's office with either a simple soft bandage or removable splint. Follow-up radiographs are unnecessary, and patients can return to activities when they are asymptomatic. Orthopedic follow-up is not needed.

Hand

Fractures of the metacarpal are commonly seen, and should be referred to an orthopedic surgeon because they often require rigid casting. Finger fractures, if minimally displaced and minimally angulated, can be treated with buddy taping. Finger fractures heal quickly in children, with resolution of symptoms with 2 to 3 weeks. Any significant deformity after taping, or any rotational deformity, should be referred to an orthopedic surgeon. Examples of phalangeal fractures of the thumb and fingers are shown in **Fig. 16**.

REFERENCES

1. Boutis K, Grootendorst P, Willan A, et al. Effect of the Low Risk Ankle Rule on the frequency of radiography in children with ankle injuries. CMAJ 2013;185:E731–8. http://dx.doi.org/10.1503/cmaj.122050.
2. Moore BR, Hampers LC, Clark KD. Performance of a decision rule for radiographs of pediatric knee injuries. J Emerg Med 2005;28:257–61. http://dx.doi.org/10.1016/j.jemermed.2004.09.010.
3. Andersen K, Jensen PO, Lauritzen J. Treatment of clavicular fractures. Figure-of-eight bandage versus a simple sling. Acta Orthop Scand 1987;58:71–4.
4. Boutis K, Unni G, Narayanan B, et al. Magnetic resonance imaging of clinically suspected Salter-Harris I fracture of the distal fibula. Injury 2010;41:852–6. http://dx.doi.org/10.1016/j.injury.2010.04.015.

5. Pandya NK, Namdari S, Hosalkar HS. Displaced clavicle fractures in adolescents: facts, controversies, and current trends. J Am Acad Orthop Surg 2012;20:498–505. http://dx.doi.org/10.5435/JAAOS-20-08-498.
6. Song KS, Kang CH, Min BW, et al. Internal oblique radiographs for diagnosis of nondisplaced or minimally displaced lateral condylar fractures of the humerus in children. J Bone Joint Surg Am 2007;89:58–63. http://dx.doi.org/10.2106/JBJS.E.01387.
7. Oakley EA, Ooi KS, Barnett PL. A randomized controlled trial of 2 methods of immobilizing torus fractures of the distal forearm. Pediatr Emerg Care 2008;24:65–70. http://dx.doi.org/10.1097/PEC.0b013e318163db13.
8. Plint AC, Perry JJ, Correll R, et al. A randomized, controlled trial of removable splinting versus casting for wrist buckle fractures in children. Pediatrics 2006;117:691–7. http://dx.doi.org/10.1542/peds.2005-0801.
9. West S, Andrews J, Bebbington A, et al. Buckle fractures of the distal radius are safely treated in a soft bandage: a randomized prospective trial of bandage versus plaster cast. J Pediatr Orthop 2005;25:322–5.

Update on Evaluation and Treatment of Scoliosis

Ron El-Hawary, MD, MSc, FRCS(C)*, Chukwudi Chukwunyerenwa, MD, MCh, FRCS(C)

KEYWORDS

• Scoliosis • Bracing • Surgery • VEPTR

KEY POINTS

- Scoliosis can arise from a variety of causes and is defined as a lateral curvature of the spine greater than 10°.
- The most common cause of scoliosis is idiopathic, which accounts for up to 80% of scoliosis in children.
- The Adam's forward bending test is a clinical evaluation of axial plane rotation that is associated with scoliosis.
- The goal of treatment is to prevent curve progression. If a curve progresses beyond 50°, it will likely continue to progress into adulthood.
- For children with early onset scoliosis, the goal of treatment is also to maintain spine, chest, and pulmonary development throughout childhood.

INTRODUCTION

Scoliosis can arise from a variety of causes and is defined as a lateral curvature of the spine greater than 10° on an anterior-posterior standing radiograph (**Fig. 1**). However, in reality, it is a 3-dimensional structural deformity that includes a curvature in the anterior-posterior plane, angulation in the sagittal plane, and rotation in the transverse plane. This 3-dimensional deformity differentiates scoliosis from nonstructural spine deformities, which arise as compensation for abnormalities in other regions (eg, lower limb disorders resulting in limb length discrepancy), in which case the deformity is mono-planer and resolves when the primary abnormality is treated.

IDIOPATHIC SCOLIOSIS

The most common cause of scoliosis is idiopathic, which accounts for up to 80% of scoliosis in children.[1] The cause of idiopathic scoliosis is unknown and is a diagnosis

Disclosures: Consulting Depuy-Synthes Spine, Medtronic Canada, Halifax Biomedical Inc, research/educational support Depuy-Synthes Spine, Medtronic Canada (R. El-Hawary). Nothing to disclose (C. Chukwunyerenwa).
Division of Orthopaedic Surgery, Department of Surgery, IWK Health Center, 5850 University Avenue, PO Box 9700, Halifax, Nova Scotia B3K-6R8, Canada
* Corresponding author.
E-mail address: ron.el-hawary@iwk.nshealth.ca

Scoliosis Classification

Neuromuscular

Neuropathic

- Upper motor neuron
  - Cerebral palsy
  - Spinocerebellar degeneration
    - Friedrich's Ataxia
    - Charcot-Marie-Tooth
    Disease

  - Syringomyelia
    - Spinal Cord Tumor
    - Spinal Cord Trauma

- Lower motor neuron
  - Poliomyelitis
  - Traumatic
  - Spinal muscular atrophy
  - Myelomeningocele

Myopathic

- Arthrogryposis
- Muscular dystrophy
  - Duchenne's
  - Limb-girdle
  - Fascioscapulohumeral
- Congenital hypotonia
- Myotonia dystrophica

Idiopathic
- Infantile
- Juvenile
- Adolescent

Congenital
- Failure of formation
  - Wedge vertebra
  - Hemivertebra
- Failure of segmentation
  - Unilateral bar
  - Block veterbra
- Mixed

Miscellaneous
- Neurofibromatosis
- Connective tissue
  - Marfan's syndrome
  - Ehlers-Danlos
- Osteochondrodystrophies
  - Diastrophic Dysplasia
  - Mucopolysaccaridosis
  - SED
  - MED
  - Achondroplasia
- Metabolic
  - Rickets
  - OI
  - Homosystinuria
- Tumors

Fig. 1. Classification of scoliosis.

of exclusion. It is classified based on age of onset into infantile (0–3 years), juvenile (3–10 years), and adolescent (>10 years).[2] These 3 periods mark the different periods of growth velocity during childhood; hence, the curves behave differently.

A different classification, first used by Dickson,[3] separates idiopathic scoliosis into early onset (<5 years) and late onset (>5 years), given that the natural history, prevalence, and treatment methods for patients with scoliosis when younger than 5 years is significantly different from patients presenting with scoliosis when older than 5 years. Another advantage of this classification is that it separates scoliosis into 2 distinct periods of pulmonary development; from 0 to 5 years of age is the period of major pulmonary development, and a thoracic deformity during this period will have a greater impact on pulmonary function than one developing in later years. Early onset scoliosis includes all patients with an age of onset of less than 5 years regardless of the cause; however, more recently, there is a growing trend toward changing this definition to less than 10 years of age regardless of cause.

Infantile Idiopathic Scoliosis

Infantile idiopathic scoliosis accounts for less than 1% of idiopathic scoliosis.[4] It is more common in boys (ratio: 3:2); most are convex left curves (75%–90%); most tend to resolve spontaneously and often can be associated with plagiocephaly (80%–90%).[5–7]

Juvenile Idiopathic Scoliosis

Juvenile idiopathic scoliosis makes up between 12% and 21% of patients with idiopathic scoliosis.[2,8,9] Juvenile idiopathic scoliosis is a transition between infantile and adolescent idiopathic scoliosis. There is a slight female preponderance ranging from 1.6:1.0 to 4.4:1.0, which tends to increase with increasing age of onset.[9,10] A right thoracic curve is predominant in this category. Because the juvenile period is a period of slow spinal growth,[11] the natural history is that of slow progression until about

10 years of age when curve progression is more rapid, coinciding with the period of accelerated spine growth.[9] Because of the earlier age of onset compared with adolescent idiopathic scoliosis, they are more likely to progress to severe deformity and less likely to respond to nonsurgical treatment.[9,10]

Adolescent Idiopathic Scoliosis

Adolescent idiopathic scoliosis (AIS) is the most common type of scoliosis with an overall incidence in the population of 2% (**Fig. 2**). The female-to-male ratio tends to increase with increasing magnitude of the curve: 1:1 for curves less than 10°, 1.4:1.0 for curves between 11° and 20°, 5.4:1.0 for curves 21° and greater, and 7.2:1.0 for curves requiring treatment.[12] The natural history and risk of progression of AIS depends on several factors, including skeletal maturity, sex, and curve magnitude. Curves in girls are more likely to progress and are more likely to require treatment. The curve magnitude increases with skeletal growth; hence, the more skeletally immature a patient is, the greater the likelihood is for the curve to progress. Another determinant of curve progression is the curve magnitude at presentation. Patients with curves greater than 20° who are skeletally immature are at a greater risk for curve progression.

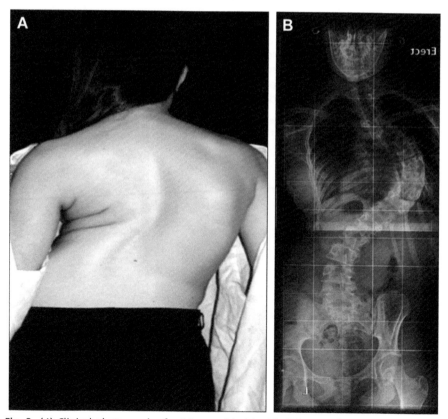

Fig. 2. (*A*) Clinical photograph of a 14-year-old girl with AIS. Note the convex right main thoracic scoliosis with resultant elevation of the right shoulder and trunk shift to the right. (*B*) Standing posteroanterior radiograph of the same patient indicating a scoliosis of greater than 90°. Radiographs are oriented as if looking at the patient from behind.

CONGENITAL SCOLIOSIS

Congenital scoliosis arises as a result of congenital malformations of the spine that are present at birth; however, because of the effects of growth, the deformity may not be apparent until later in childhood. Congenital scoliosis is classified as a failure of formation of a vertebral body (hemivertebrae), failure of segmentation between 2 or more vertebrae (bar), or a failure of segmentation in combination with a failure of formation (**Fig. 3**). The natural history of congenital scoliosis depends on the type of malformation, with the combination of a unilateral hemivertebrae and a contralateral bar having the worst prognosis.[13] A significant percentage (61%) of patients with congenital scoliosis have an associated anomaly in other organ systems, which may appear independently or as part of a syndrome. VACTERL syndrome (vertebral, anorectal, cardiac, tracheoesophageal, renal, and limb) is often found to be associated with congenital scoliosis.[14–16] It is important to screen for these other potential abnormalities when assessing patients with congenital scoliosis. The authors routinely order renal ultrasound and echocardiograms on all patients with a diagnosis of congenital scoliosis.

NEUROMUSCULAR SCOLIOSIS

Neuromuscular scoliosis is scoliosis arising as a result of neurologic or muscular disorders. The Scoliosis Research Society has classified it into neuropathic and myopathic causes. Neuropathic causes include upper motor neuron lesions, such as cerebral palsy, spinocerebellar degeneration (Fredrick ataxia, Charcot-Marie-Tooth disease), syringomyelia, spinal cord tumors and trauma, and lower motor neuron lesions, such as poliomyelitis, spinal muscular atrophy, and myelomeningocele. Myopathic conditions include arthrogryposis, muscular dystrophies (Duchene,

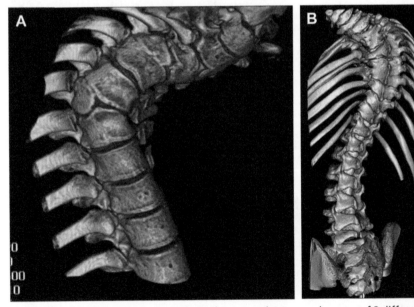

Fig. 3. Three-dimensional reconstructions of computed tomography scans of 2 different patients with congenital scoliosis. (*A*) There is a failure of formation with a hemivertebrae visualized at the apex of deformity. (*B*) There is a failure of segmentation with unilateral bar and fused ribs at the apex of deformity.

limb-girdle, facioscapulohumeral), congenital hypotonia, and myotonia dystrophica. The underlying cause for all neuromuscular scoliosis is the lack of muscular support to the spinal column, which allows gravity and posturing that leads to deformity of the spine. The age of onset of neuromuscular scoliosis and the natural history vary depending on the cause.

MISCELLANEOUS CAUSES

Other causes of scoliosis include tumors, neurofibromatosis, connective tissue disorders (Marfan syndrome, Ehlers-Danlos syndrome), osteochondrodystrophies (dystrophic dysplasia, mucopolysaccharidosis, spondyloepiphyseal dysplasia, multiple epiphyseal dysplasia, achondroplasia), and metabolic causes (rickets, osteogenesis imperfecta).

EVALUATION OF SCOLIOSIS

The evaluation of patients with scoliosis starts with a detailed history and thorough physical examination, which are aimed at identifying nonidiopathic causes and at identifying features that are associated with rapid progression of the scoliosis.

HISTORY

Keys in the history include the age of onset, history of progression of the spinal deformity, and how the curve was noticed and by whom (child, parent, school screening, or by the primary physician). The usual presenting complaint is chest wall or back asymmetry. Adolescent girls will sometimes complain of breast asymmetry, unequal shoulders, uneven waistline and difficulty with fitting clothes.

Associated symptoms, such as pain, neurologic, or respiratory, should be sought. Although pain is not a prominent feature of scoliosis, about one-quarter of patients with AIS will present with pain,[17] which is mostly benign and nonspecific. Some patients will complain of posterior chest wall pain around the area of rib prominence. Persistent and severe back pain, with red flags signs like fever and constitutional symptoms, might be related to infection and should be investigated further. Back pain that is worse at night and relieved by nonsteroidal antiinflammatory medication might suggest osteoid osteoma of the spine, which may create a deformity of the spine.

History of breathing difficulty and failure to thrive in a child presenting with scoliosis and chest wall deformity might suggest pulmonary insufficiency syndrome and warrants further pulmonary evaluation.

The evaluating physician should seek to identify neurologic symptoms, such as sensory or motor weakness and difficulty with coordination, gait, and balance. Any bowel or bladder symptoms may be secondary to intraspinal diagnoses like syringomyelia, tumor or tethered cord.

For a child presenting with scoliosis, a detailed perinatal history including any illness during the pregnancy, medications taken, length of gestation, mode of delivery, and birth weight should be obtained. Developmental history, both motor and cognition, should also be noted as these may indicate a neuromuscular or syndromic causes of scoliosis.

For adolescent patients, a history of adolescent growth spurts and other maturity indicators like menarche status in girls (both onset and duration) are important. The risk of curve progression and methods of treatment depend on the amount of spinal growth remaining. Psychosocial history is important in assessing an adolescent with scoliosis, as patients are often not happy with the cosmetic deformity. The patients' main desire to treat the scoliosis may be related to the cosmetic deformity.

Past medical and surgical history are important in ruling out any syndromic features. A history of heart disease might prompt one to look at other syndromic features (Marfan syndrome, for example). Any family history of scoliosis should be noted, as there is often a genetic component associated with AIS.[18] For neuromuscular patients, it is important to note the associated comorbidities, including medications that could impact any planned surgical treatment.

EXAMINATION

The physical examination should include a general head-to-toe examination, including assessment for pubertal development in adolescents. Patients' height should be documented and plotted on a growth chart to monitor for peak growth velocity. Clinicians should evaluate for syndromic features and associated deformities: The presence of plagiocephaly, bat ear, or torticollis may suggest infantile idiopathic scoliosis; skin manifestations, such as café au lait spots and axillary freckles, may suggest neurofibromatosis; sacral dimple, hairy patch, or lipoma at the lower back may suggest spinal dysraphism (ie, myelomeningocele); cavus foot may suggest a sensory-motor abnormality (ie, Charcot-Marie-Tooth Disease or a spinal cord tumor). Tall patients, with an increased ratio of arm span to height, should prompt examination for other features of Marfan syndrome, including cardiac and ophthalmologic examination. The presence of joint hyperlaxity and poor skin tone might point to a connective tissue disorder, such as Ehlers-Danlos syndrome.

Examination of the deformity begins with inspection (from behind the patients) for shoulder and flank asymmetry. Care should be taken to ensure that the pelvis is as level as possible. If the pelvis remains unlevel, this might suggest a leg-length discrepancy, which may be the cause of the scoliosis. If this seems to be the case, the patients should be examined while in the seated position. A curve that is caused by a leg-length discrepancy disappears with patients sitting.

The Adam's forward bending test assesses the curve rotation (**Fig. 4**).[19,20] By assessing patients from behind, while they forward flex, the axial plane rotation associated with a structural scoliosis will be evidenced by a rib prominence in the thoracic spine and/or paraspinal muscle prominence in the lumbar spine. In a child that is too young for an Adam's forward bending test, laying the child prone may help in assessing the rotational deformity. The curve flexibility can be assessed at the same time by rotating the child to a lateral position while still supine. Suspending the child under the arm of the examiner can also assess the flexibility of the spinal deformity. Also, an evaluation for asymmetry or limitation in chest excursion, may suggest thoracic insufficiency syndrome.

The clinician should perform a complete neurologic examination including a cranial nerve examination as well as sensory, motor, and reflex evaluation of the upper and lower extremities. The abdominal reflex should be performed in order to evaluate for potential neural axis abnormalities in the thoracic spine. Absent abdominal reflex is also seen in some patients with Chiari malformation.[21]

SCREENING FOR ADOLESCENT IDIOPATHIC SCOLIOSIS

School screening of healthy asymptomatic adolescents for AIS has been a controversial issue over the years, with arguments for and against the benefit of routine screening. However, the Scoliosis Research Society, the Pediatric Orthopedic Society of North America, the American Academy of Orthopedic Surgeons, and the

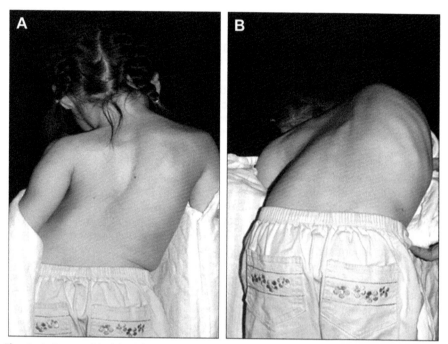

Fig. 4. A 7-year-old girl with congenital scoliosis. (*A*) Standing evaluation evaluates the lateral curvature of the spine. (*B*) Adam's forward bending test evaluates the axial plane rotation of the spine. This patient's preoperative and postoperative computed tomography scans are demonstrated in **Figs. 3**B and **10**B, respectively.

American Academy of Pediatrics all agree that girls should be screened twice, at 10 and 12 years of age, whereas boys should be screened once at 13 or 14 years of age.[22] Clinical signs used in screening programs include shoulder asymmetry, asymmetry of scapular prominence, greater space between the arm and the body on one side compared with the opposite side with arm hanging loosely by the side, head not centered over the pelvis (examining patients from the back), and the Adam's forward bending test. A scoliometer is used to measure any rotational deformity on the Adam's forward bending test, and a trunk rotation of 7° or greater is an indication for referral. Modern scoliometers are now readily available as applications for smart phones. The clinical benefit of screening is thought to be that it leads to the early detection of curves, and the institution of early brace therapy can alter the natural history of the deformity.

RADIOGRAPHIC EVALUATION
Plain Radiograph

Initial radiographic evaluation of patients with suspected scoliosis is with a standing posterior-anterior (PA) and lateral radiograph of the whole spine include the hip joints in a single 3-ft film (see **Fig. 2**B). PA radiography minimizes radiation to organs including the breast and thyroid. Recently, a low dose radiographic system has been introduced (EOS Imaging, Paris, France), which can capture these images of standing patients in a single scan in both frontal and sagittal views simultaneously without having to stitch the images together and without vertical distortion.[23] If there is an associated leg-length discrepancy, it should be corrected by placing an appropriately sized wooden block under the short leg to level the pelvis while the standing radiographs are obtained. A supine radiograph is obtained if a patient is too young to stand independently, and a sitting radiograph is obtained for wheelchair ambulators.

PA radiographs are conventionally viewed with the heart on the left side as if looking at patients from behind. This position mimics the view that the clinician has during the clinical assessment for scoliosis and is also the position of patients during posterior spinal fusion and instrumentation surgery for scoliosis. In addition to evaluating the curve magnitudes by measuring the Cobb angles, look for any obvious vertebral or rib malformations, which could suggest congenital scoliosis. The curves are described by the direction of the convexity and the location of the apex. For instance, most AIS curves are right main thoracic curves (see **Fig. 2B**).

On the lateral radiograph, there is generally apical hypokyphosis associated with idiopathic scoliosis. Lack of vertebral rotation or lack of hypokyphosis at the apex may suggest a nonidiopathic cause of the deformity, such as tumor (osteoid osteoma) or intraspinal abnormality (syringomyelia). For patients with AIS, examine for features of skeletal maturity, including the Risser sign (maturity of iliac crest apophysis) and open versus closed triradiate cartilage of the acetabulum. These features are used in predicting the growth remaining, hence, the curve progression, which influences the choice of treatment. The curve magnitude is evaluated using the Cobb method of measuring the angular deformity from the upper end vertebrae to the lower end vertebrae.

For patients with infantile idiopathic scoliosis, the likelihood of curve progression is determined radiographically by measuring the rib-vertebral angle difference (RVAD) of Mehta (**Fig. 5**).[24] An RVAD of 20° or less indicates that the curve is unlikely to progress, whereas an RVAD of 20° or more indicates a curve is likely to progress.

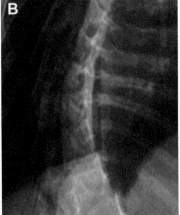

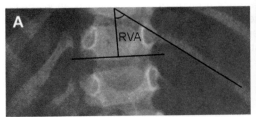

Fig. 5. Two methods of determining risk of scoliosis curve progression in patients with infantile idiopathic scoliosis. (*A*) Evaluation of the rib vertebral angle. At the apex of deformity, draw a line along the end plate of the vertebrae. Draw another line perpendicular to the first line. Draw a line along the rib. Measure the angle between the second and third lines. Repeat this for the contralateral rib. The difference between the 2 angles is the RVAD. If the RVAD is greater than 20°, this indicates significant rotation of the scoliosis and a high likelihood of curve progression. (*B*) Example of a phase-2 rib head. It also indicates significant rotation of the scoliosis and a high likelihood of curve progression. RVA, rib vertebral angle.

An additional method of predicting curve progression also described by Mehta[24] is the relationship of the convex rib head with the apical vertebra body (phase of the rib head). In phase-1 rib, there is no overlap of the rib head of the convex rib of the apical vertebra with the vertebral body; such curves have a low risk of progression. However, in phase-2 rib, there is an overlap; hence, there is a high risk of progression (see **Fig. 5**).[24]

ANCILLARY INVESTIGATION

These tests are recommended for further evaluation of scoliosis and to help with surgical planning.

Computed Tomography Scan

A computed tomography (CT) scan may be used to further define the anatomy, including assessing congenital abnormalities or investigating for suspected tumor cause. CT can also be used in evaluating 3-dimensioinal lung volume in young patients who may not be able to comply with pulmonary function testing. Supine bending and stretch radiographs are used to assess the flexibility of the curve.

MRI

MRI is indicated for all patients presenting with early onset scoliosis. It is not routinely performed for patients with AIS, except for those with pain, atypical curve pattern (**Fig. 6**), large curve on presentation, rapidly progressive curve, or for patients with abnormal neurologic examination. There is an increasing trend to obtain an MRI scan for any patient requiring operative treatment of their scoliosis to rule out any unexpected intraspinal abnormality (see **Fig. 6**).

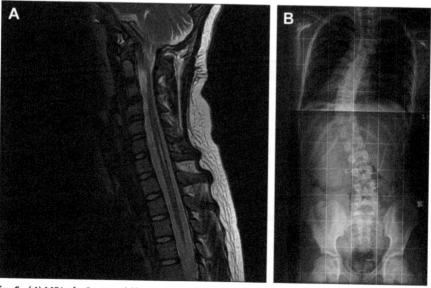

Fig. 6. (*A*) MRI of a 9-year-old boy with scoliosis. The sagittal plane image demonstrates associated Chiari malformation and resultant cervical syrinx. (*B*) PA radiograph of the same patient demonstrating a left main thoracic curve pattern. This atypical curve pattern has a higher rate of associated neural axis abnormality and is an indication to obtain an MRI.

Other Investigations

Other investigations that are useful for a preoperative workup include an echocardiogram and a renal ultrasound for patients with congenital scoliosis; assessment of pulmonary function in patients with early onset scoliosis; and assessment of overall nutritional status, especially for patients with neurologic disorders.

MANAGEMENT OF SCOLIOSIS
Management of Adolescent Idiopathic Scoliosis

Because the natural history of AIS at skeletal maturity is for continued progression of the curve into adulthood only if the deformity is greater than 50°, the ultimate goal of the treatment of AIS is to keep the scoliosis less than 50° at maturity. The treatment choices are based on several factors, including curve magnitude, type and location of the curve, level of maturity, remaining growth, cosmetic appearance, and patient psychosocial factors. The options include observation, bracing, and surgery. In broad terms, the treatment guidelines for AIS are as follows:

Observation

Observation is recommended for curves that are 25° or less, regardless of the level of skeletal maturity. These patients require close radiographic monitoring for evidence of curve progression (5°–6° change in Cobb angle). The follow-up interval should be 3 to 6 months depending on the size of the curve and the level of skeletal maturity. Patients who are Risser grade 0 or 1 (immature) with curves close to 25° should be seen more frequently (3 monthly), whereas those who are Risser 3 and greater (more mature) with curves that are 20° or less are seen every 6 months.

Brace

Brace treatment is recommended for patients with curves between 25° and 45° who are Risser 2 or less. The goal of bracing is to prevent curve progression and to keep it below the surgical range at skeletal maturity. The most common type of brace used currently is the thoracolumbosacral orthosis (TLSO), which includes the Boston (**Fig. 7**), Charleston, and Providence braces. These braces are only suitable for curves with an apex at T7 or lower. The specific indication for the brace type depends on the type of curve. For the brace treatment to be successful, patients must be willing to comply with the prescribed amount of time in the brace. A recent randomized controlled trial by Weinstein and colleagues[25] demonstrates that brace treatment was effective in decreasing the curve progression to the surgical threshold in AIS. They also showed that the benefit of brace wear increases with longer hours of wear. Patients should also be willing to accept their cosmetic deformity before treatment, as this is unlikely to improve. Hence, careful patient counseling before bracing is important.

Surgical treatment

Surgical treatment is recommended for patients with curves greater than 45° who are Risser 2 or less or for curves greater than 50 who are Risser 3 and greater. The goal of surgical treatment is to arrest the curve progression while improving spinal balance and alignment. This goal is achieved by inducing fusion of the spine by way of instrumentation and bone grafting. Fusion techniques have evolved over the years from Harrington's[26] introduction of the hook and rod construct in the 1960s to Luque's[27] segmental fixation with wires and the current third-generation segmental fixation with pedicle screws (**Fig. 8**). The underlying principle of all fixation techniques involves the placement of bony anchors, including hooks, wires, or pedicle screws to the

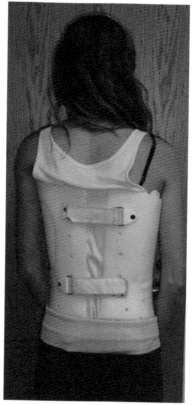

Fig. 7. A patient with AIS who is being treated with a TLSO.

vertebrae and connecting them to a dual rod construct. Fusion can be performed anteriorly, posteriorly, or both depending on the curve type, magnitude, skeletal maturity, and the available skill set of the surgeon. The factors to consider in preoperative planning include the curve type and magnitude, spinal balance, curve flexibility, and the level of skeletal maturity.

Management of Early Onset Scoliosis

Recently, there has been a realization that regardless of cause, young patients with scoliosis have an increase risk of developing a pulmonary insufficiency syndrome that can lead to increased morbidity and mortality. This increased risk is because the bronchial tree and the alveolar are only fully developed by 8 years of age and the thoracic cavity is 50% of adult volume by 10 years of age.[28,29] Also, the spine has its most rapid growth during the first 5 years of life (2.2 cm/y) before it slows down during the following 5 years (0.9 cm/y) and peaks again at puberty (1.8 cm/y).[30] It has been shown that gaining a thoracic height of least 18 cm at maturity is associated with a better pulmonary function.[31] These factors are important to consider in the treatment of early onset scoliosis. The goal of the treatment of early onset scoliosis is not only to stop progression of the spine deformity but to also allow for continued growth and development of the spine, thoracic cavity, and lungs. The treatment options include observation, nonsurgical treatment (bracing, casting, halo traction), and growth-friendly surgery.

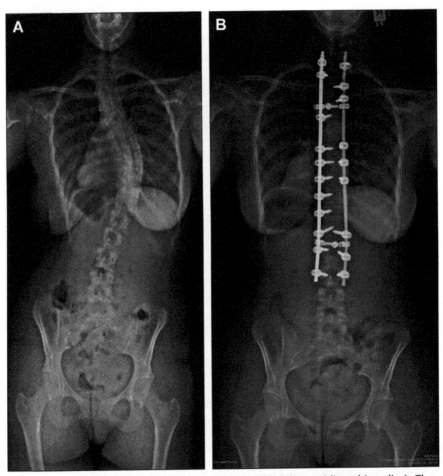

Fig. 8. Standing PA radiographs of a 16-year-old girl with adolescent idiopathic scoliosis. These radiographs were obtained with a low dose radiographic system (EOS Imaging, Paris, France), which has significantly less radiation dose as compared with conventional radiography. (*A*) Preoperative radiographs demonstrating a right main thoracic scoliosis greater than 50°. (*B*) Radiographs obtained after posterior spinal fusion and instrumentation surgery.

Observation
Observation is for patients whose curves have a low risk of progression based on Mehta's criteria. These curves have a curve angle of 25° or less and an RVAD of 20° or less and are followed up with serial radiographs every 4 to 6 months. Treatment should be commenced if there is curve progression of 10° or more. Curves with an RVAD of 20° or more or a phase-2 rib relationship are likely to progress and require treatment.

Serial casting
Serial casting is one of the nonsurgical methods used to delay fusion surgery in patients with early onset scoliosis (**Fig. 9**). It has been shown to be a viable alternative to growth-friendly surgery in early onset scoliosis[32] and has been shown to cure some small idiopathic curves.[33] Its attractiveness is that it is a nonsurgical treatment, hence, avoiding the potential complications with surgical treatment; however, patients

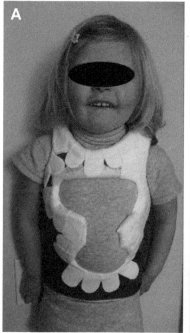 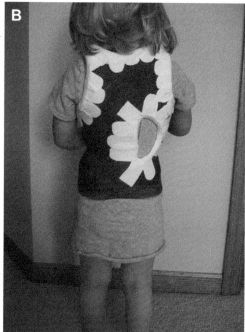

Fig. 9. A patient with early onset scoliosis who is being treated with a derotation cast. (*A*) Note the anterior chest and abdominal windows to allow for chest wall and abdominal excursion during respiration. (*B*) Viewed from behind, a window along the concavity of the scoliosis allows for the deformity to derotate in the axial plane. (*Courtesy of* J. d'Astous, MD, Salt Lake City, Utah, USA.)

still require general anesthetics for its application and during routine cast changes every 3 to 4 months. There has been a recent increase in the use of casting in the management of early onset scoliosis with the realization of the high complication rate associated with growth-friendly surgical techniques (spinal growing rods and rib-based distraction surgery). It is indicated for patients with documented curve progression of 10° or greater, patients with curves of 25° or greater at presentation, those with an RVAD of 20° or greater or phase-2 rib rotation. Casting may be poorly tolerated in patients with poor pulmonary function or those with a neuromuscular disorder.

Bracing
Bracing is another nonsurgical method of delaying a curve. Bracing is an alternative to serial casting in patients who cannot tolerate casting and can also be used as a step down from casting after a satisfactory improvement in the curve with casting. It has an advantage over casting in that it is removable; however, this may contribute to lack of compliance in patients treated with a brace.

Surgery
Surgery is indicated for patients with progressive deformity or when casting/bracing has been ineffective or are contraindicated. Historically, surgical treatment of progressive early onset scoliosis has been spinal fusion similar to those performed in adolescence. Unfortunately, early surgical fusion ultimately led to restrictive lung disease because of the lack of growth of the spine and the pulmonary system, which resulted in early mortality from pulmonary insufficiency syndrome.[31,34,35] These outcomes

have led to a shift toward growth-friendly surgery with the goal of arresting curve progression while allowing for spine growth and pulmonary development.

Several growth-friendly surgical techniques have been developed over the years. Currently, the most commonly used technique is that of posterior distraction-based surgeries, which can be either spine based or rib based (**Fig. 10**). Spine-based distraction (spinal growing rods) involves the placement of anchors in the spine proximal and distal to the curve, which are connected to 2 rods. Rib-based distractions are similar to spine-based distraction; however, the proximal anchors are attached to ribs. The curve is controlled by serial distraction procedures approximately every 6 months, which grows the spine through the unfused segment. VEPTR is more commonly used in patients with associated chest wall deformity, such as absent or fused ribs. Given that posterior distraction treatment requires repetitive surgical interventions, the complication rates are high. Although these complications are a relative improvement as compared with the grim natural history of early onset scoliosis and to the poor long-term pulmonary outcomes associated with early surgical fusion, the quest for newer surgical techniques that do not require repetitive surgical interventions continues.

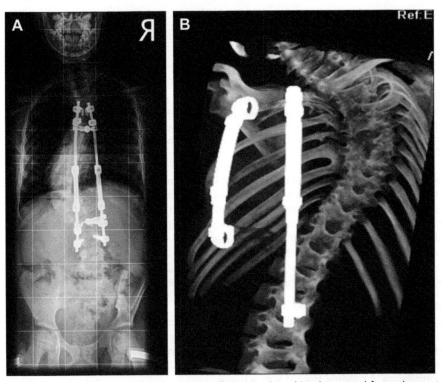

Fig. 10. Radiographic examples of posterior distraction based implants used for early onset scoliosis. (*A*) Image of an 8-year-old boy with juvenile idiopathic scoliosis who was treated with spinal growing rods. Note the superior and inferior foundations of spinal implants, which anchor the dual telescopic growing rods. (*B*) Three-dimensional CT reconstruction of the 7-year-old girl with congenital scoliosis and fused ribs who is featured clinically in **Fig. 4**. She has been treated with a rib-based distraction surgery, which is anchored to the ribs as well as to the spine. This type of device works well if there is an associated chest wall deformity. Note the improved spread between her left-sided ribs as compared with her preoperative CT scan demonstrated in **Fig. 3B**.

One such technique, still in its infancy, is growth guidance surgery (Shilla and Luque trolley systems), which involves a limited fusion at the apex of the curve with rods that are linked to anchors proximal and distal to the curve (**Fig. 11**). Because the rods are not completely constrained by the proximal and distal anchors, the rods are able to glide along the spine, which allows for continued spinal growth without periodic distraction surgeries. A variation on this theme is the magnetically controlled growing rod. This technique is similar to the commonly used spinal growing rods; however, rather than periodic distraction surgeries to lengthen the rods, the rods can be lengthened with the application of an external magnet in the clinic environment.

Another new technique that is evolving is convex side growth inhibition (staples and tethers). This technique involves applying a compression device on the convex side of the curve, producing inhibition of spine growth on that side and allowing the concave site to continue to grow, thereby strengthening the spine over time (**Fig. 12**). The advantage of this technique is also the avoidance of frequent anesthesia for distraction surgeries.

Management of Neuromuscular Scoliosis

Neuromuscular scoliosis includes a heterogeneous group of patients with different multisystem involvement; therefore, the treatment varies with the individual condition. In general, most patients with neuromuscular scoliosis are nonambulatory and are

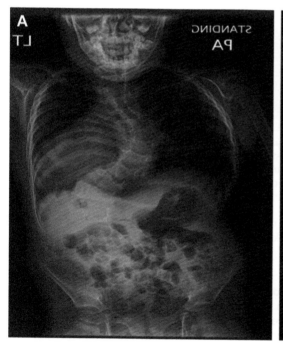
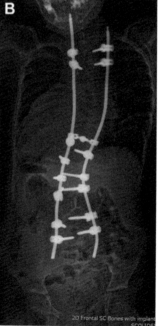

Fig. 11. Radiographs of a 6-year-old boy with syndromic scoliosis (Marfan). (*A*) Preoperative radiographs demonstrate significant thoracic and lumbar scoliosis. (*B*) Radiographs obtained after a growth guidance procedure. Note the anchors at the apex of deformity as well as at the superior and inferior ends of the constructs. The anchors at the upper and lower ends of the rods are designed in a way that they allow for the patient's spine to continue to grow along the rods, which are purposefully left long to allow for this.

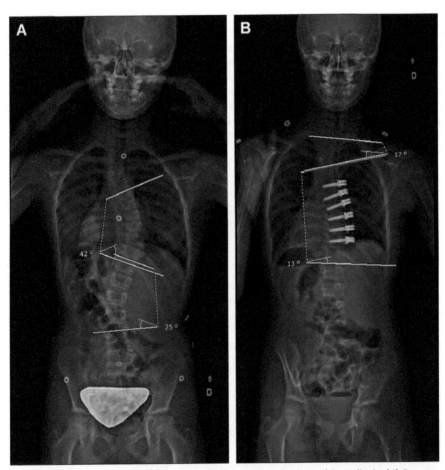

Fig. 12. Radiographs of a skeletally immature patient with idiopathic scoliosis. (*A*) Preoperative image demonstrates a modest right main thoracic scoliosis. (*B*) Radiograph obtained after convex growth inhibition surgery using a (radiolucent) polyethylene tether that is anchored by thoracoscopically placed vertebral body screws. (*Courtesy of* S. Parent, MD, Montreal, Quebec, Canada.)

wheelchair ambulators. The goal of treatment is to obtain a balanced spine over a level pelvis in order to maintain wheelchair seating balance.

Nonsurgical treatment
Nonsurgical treatments include wheelchair modification and bracing. These treatments can be technically demanding and require an experienced wheelchair specialist and orthotics department. Brace treatment is less effective in neuromuscular patients than in patients with AIS; however, the goal of brace treatment in neuromuscular patients is not to stop curve progression as in AIS but rather to maintain an upright posture in their wheelchair.

Surgical treatment
Surgical treatment and indications vary depending on the type of condition. For patients with cerebral palsy, most surgeons will consider surgery for a progressive curve of 50° or greater or when there is deterioration in functional sitting. Other factors, like

medical comorbidity and caretaker concerns, should be taken into consideration. In patients with Duchene muscular dystrophy, surgery is advocated once the curve is more than the 20° to 30° range in nonambulatory patients because the natural history is that of rapid curve progression once patients are nonambulatory. In addition, the pulmonary and cardiac function of these patients generally worsens over time. There is increased surgical complication in patients with neuromuscular scoliosis; hence, a thorough preoperative workup and optimization is essential for these patients.

In terms of surgical planning, factors to consider include fusion levels, fixation type, and approach (anterior, posterior, or both). Most neuromuscular patients require long fusion from T2 to the pelvis (**Fig. 13**). Fixation to T2 is necessary to prevent proximal

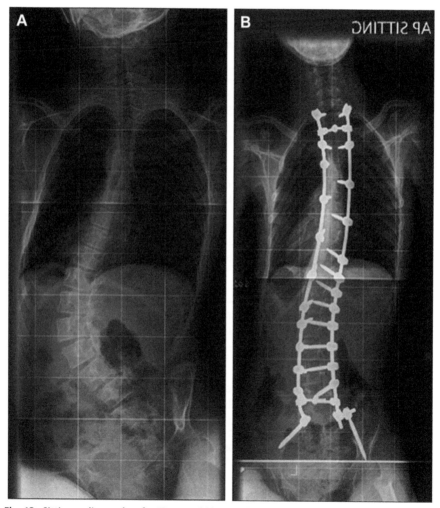

Fig. 13. Sitting radiographs of a 13-year-old boy with scoliosis secondary to a neuromuscular condition (cerebral palsy). (*A*) Preoperative images demonstrate the typical neuromuscular curve pattern with a long thoracolumbar scoliosis extending to the pelvis with a resultant pelvic obliquity. (*B*) Radiograph obtained after posterior spinal fusion and instrumentation surgery. Note the extension of the implants to include the pelvis, which allows for correction of pelvic obliquity, which should improve wheelchair sitting balance.

junctional problems like kyphosis and screw pullout, whereas fixation to the pelvis is necessary to address pelvic obliquity that is often associated with neuromuscular curves. The exception to this is in ambulatory patients whereby pelvic fixation is thought to impair the ability to ambulate. Because of a combination of a high pseudoarthrosis rate and osteoporotic bone in these patients, segmental fixation is required. The choice of instrumentation depends on the surgeon's preference, ranging from pedicle screw fixation to a hybrid of screws, wires, and hooks.

SUMMARY

Scoliosis is a 3-dimensional structural deformity of the spine. Although the causes are many, most patients have idiopathic scoliosis. A thorough clinical assessment and radiological evaluation is required to identify the nonidiopathic causes and to institute appropriate treatment. The treatment of scoliosis varies depending on the cause and ranges from observation, bracing, and casting to surgery.

REFERENCES

1. The Terminology Committee of the Scoliosis Research Society. A glossary of scoliosis terms. Spine 1976;1(1):57–8.
2. James JI. Idiopathic scoliosis. J Bone Joint Surg Br 1954;36B(1):36–49.
3. Dickson RA. Conservative treatment for idiopathic scoliosis. J Bone Joint Surg Br 1985;67(2):176–81.
4. Riseborough EJ, Wynne-Davies R. A genetic survey of idiopathic scoliosis in Boston, Massachusetts. J Bone Joint Surg Am 1973;55(5):974–82.
5. James JI, Lloyd-Roberts GC, Pilcher MF. Infantile structural scoliosis. J Bone Joint Surg Br 1959;41-B:719–35.
6. Wynne-Davies R. Infantile idiopathic scoliosis. Causative factors, particularly in the first six months of life. J Bone Joint Surg Br 1975;57(2):138–41.
7. Lloyd-Roberts GC, Pilcher MF. Structural idiopathic scoliosis in infancy: a study of the natural history of 100 patients. J Bone Joint Surg Br 1965;47:520–3.
8. Ponseti IV, Friedman B. Prognosis in idiopathic scoliosis. J Bone Joint Surg Am 1950;32A(2):381–95.
9. Robinson CM, McMaster MJ. Juvenile idiopathic scoliosis. Curve patterns and prognosis in one hundred and nine patients. J Bone Joint Surg Am 1996;78(8):1140–8.
10. Figueiredo UM, James JI. Juvenile idiopathic scoliosis. J Bone Joint Surg Br 1981;63-B(1):61–6.
11. Pehrsson K, Larsson S, Oden A, et al. Long-term follow-up of patients with untreated scoliosis. A study of mortality, causes of death, and symptoms. Spine 1992;17(9):1091–6.
12. Rogala EJ, Drummond DS, Gurr J. Scoliosis: incidence and natural history. A prospective epidemiological study. J Bone Joint Surg Am 1978;60(2):173–6.
13. McMaster MJ, Ohtsuka K. The natural history of congenital scoliosis. A study of two hundred and fifty-one patients. J Bone Joint Surg Am 1982;64(8):1128–47.
14. MacEwen GD, Winter RB, Hardy JH. Evaluation of kidney anomalies in congenital scoliosis. J Bone Joint Surg Am 1972;54(7):1451–4.
15. Rittler M, Paz JE, Castilla EE. VACTERL association, epidemiologic definition and delineation. Am J Med Genet 1996;63(4):529–36. http://dx.doi.org/10.1002/(SICI)1096-8628(19960628)63:4<529::AID-AJMG4>3.0.CO;2-J.
16. Beals RK, Robbins JR, Rolfe B. Anomalies associated with vertebral malformations. Spine 1993;18(10):1329–32.

17. Ramirez N, Johnston CE, Brodeur AE. The prevalence of back pain in children who have idiopathic scoliosis. J Bone Joint Surg Am 1997;79(3):364–8.
18. Wynne-Davies R. Familial (idiopathic) scoliosis. J Bone Joint Surg Br 1998;50 B(1):24–30.
19. Adams W. Lectures on the Pathology and Treatment of Lateral and Other Forms of Curvature of the Spine, 2nd edition. London: J & A Churchill; 1882.
20. Herring JA. Tachdjian's pediatric orthopaedics. Philadelphia: Elsevier Health Sciences; 2013.
21. Muhonen MG, Menezes AH, Sawin PD, et al. Scoliosis in pediatric Chiari malformations without myelodysplasia. J Neurosurg 1992;77(1):69–77. http://dx.doi.org/10.3171/jns.1992.77.1.0069.
22. Labelle H, Richards SB, De Kleuver M, et al. Screening for adolescent idiopathic scoliosis: an information statement by the scoliosis research society international task force. Scoliosis 2013;8(1):17. http://dx.doi.org/10.1186/1748-7161-8-17.
23. Escott BG, Ravi B, Weathermon AC, et al. EOS low-dose radiography: a reliable and accurate upright assessment of lower-limb lengths. J Bone Joint Surg Am 2013;95(23):e1831–7. http://dx.doi.org/10.1016/S0021-9355(13)73964-X.
24. Mehta MH. The rib-vertebra angle in the early diagnosis between resolving and progressive infantile scoliosis. J Bone Joint Surg Br 1972;54(2):230–43.
25. Weinstein SL, Dolan LA, Wright JG, et al. Effects of bracing in adolescents with idiopathic scoliosis. N Engl J Med 2013;369(16):1512–21. http://dx.doi.org/10.1056/NEJMoa1307337.
26. Harrington PR. Treatment of scoliosis. Correction and internal fixation by spine instrumentation. J Bone Joint Surg Am 1962;44-A:591–610.
27. Luque ER. Segmental spinal instrumentation for correction of scoliosis. Clin Orthop Relat Res 1982;(163):192–8.
28. Davies G, Reid L. Growth of the alveoli and pulmonary arteries in childhood. Thorax 1970;25(6):669–81.
29. Thurlbeck WM. Postnatal human lung growth. Thorax 1982;37(8):564–71.
30. Canavese F, Dimeglio A. Normal and abnormal spine and thoracic cage development. World J Orthop 2013;4(4):167–74. http://dx.doi.org/10.5312/wjo.v4.i4.167.
31. Karol LA, Johnston C, Mladenov K, et al. Pulmonary function following early thoracic fusion in non-neuromuscular scoliosis. J Bone Joint Surg Am 2008;90(6):1272–81. http://dx.doi.org/10.2106/JBJS.G.00184.
32. Fletcher ND, McClung A, Rathjen KE, et al. Serial casting as a delay tactic in the treatment of moderate-to-severe early-onset scoliosis. J Pediatr Orthop 2012;32(7):664–71. http://dx.doi.org/10.1097/BPO.0b013e31824bdb55.
33. Mehta MH. Growth as a corrective force in the early treatment of progressive infantile scoliosis. J Bone Joint Surg Br 2005;87(9):1237–47. http://dx.doi.org/10.1302/0301-620X.87B9.16124.
34. Goldberg CJ, Gillic I, Connaughton O, et al. Respiratory function and cosmesis at maturity in infantile-onset scoliosis. Spine 2003;28(20):2397–406. http://dx.doi.org/10.1097/01.BRS.0000085367.24266.CA.
35. Vitale MG, Matsumoto H, Bye MR, et al. A retrospective cohort study of pulmonary function, radiographic measures, and quality of life in children with congenital scoliosis: an evaluation of patient outcomes after early spinal fusion. Spine 2008;33(11):1242–9. http://dx.doi.org/10.1097/BRS.0b013e3181714536.

Update on the Evaluation and Treatment of Osteogenesis Imperfecta

Jennifer Harrington, MBBS, FRACP[a], Etienne Sochett, MB ChB, FRCPC[a], Andrew Howard, MD, MSc, FRCSC[b],*

KEYWORDS

• Osteogenesis imperfecta • Collagen • Fractures • Bisphosphonates

KEY POINTS

• Osteogenesis imperfecta (OI) is the most common cause of primary osteoporosis in children and presents with variable severity.
• Ninety percent of cases of OI are due to autosomal dominant mutations of type 1 collagen genes, but new genes involved with post-translational collagen modification have been recently implicated in rare recessive forms.
• Management of children with moderate to severe OI involves physiotherapy, rehabilitation, orthopedic surgery, and consideration of bisphosphonate treatment.
• Fracture management emphasizes minimizing time and extent of immobilization to minimize secondary disuse osteoporosis. Surgical management of long bone fractures and deformities includes intramedullary fixation devices.
• Bisphosphonate therapy can increase bone mineral density and decrease bone pain and fracture incidence. The optimal treatment regimen and duration is unknown.

Osteogenesis imperfecta (OI) is a term used to describe a group of inherited connective tissue conditions that are characterized by increased bone fragility and low bone mass. With an estimated prevalence of 1 in 12,000 to 15, 000 children,[1,2] it has a broad clinical phenotype, ranging in severity from perinatal lethality to mild clinical forms without fractures. Wormian bones are present in the skull in approximately 60% of patients (**Fig. 1**).[3] Other clinical characteristics such as blue sclera, dental abnormalities, skin hyperlaxity, and joint hypermobility are heterogeneous in presentation even in affected members of the same family.

No external funding was secured for this study. The authors have no financial relationships or conflict of interests relevant to this article to disclose.
[a] Division of Endocrinology, Department of Pediatrics, Hospital for Sick Children, University of Toronto, 555 University Avenue, Toronto, Ontario M5G1X8, Canada; [b] Division of Orthopedic Surgery, Department of Pediatrics, Hospital for Sick Children, University of Toronto, 555 University Avenue, Toronto, Ontario M5G1X8, Canada
* Corresponding author.
E-mail address: andrew.howard@sickkids.ca

Pediatr Clin N Am 61 (2014) 1243–1257
http://dx.doi.org/10.1016/j.pcl.2014.08.010
0031-3955/14/$ – see front matter © 2014 Elsevier Inc. All rights reserved.

pediatric.theclinics.com

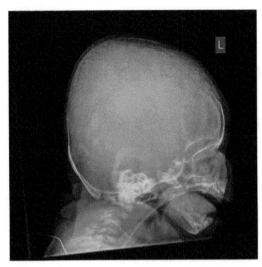

Fig. 1. Wormian bone.

Most of the cases are associated with mutations in 1 of 2 genes that encode the alpha chains of collagen type I (COL1A1 and COL1A2). Over the past 10 years, multiple additional genes involved with post-translational modification of type 1 collagen, bone cell signaling, or regulation of bone matrix homeostasis have been identified, expanding the genetic spectrum of OI.

CLASSIFICATION OF OSTEOGENESIS IMPERFECTA

The Sillence classification, published in 1979, was the first systemic classification of OI phenotype, divided based on clinical and radiographic criteria.[4] Patients were classified as having mild nondeforming (type I), moderate (type IV), severe progressively deforming (type III), or perinatal lethal (type II) OI. With increased awareness of the genetic complexity of OI and the phenotypic variability arising from mutations at single loci, there is ongoing debate about the optimal method to categorize patients. **Tables 1** and **2** outline the current known genetic mutations associated with OI. Careful analysis of the inheritance pattern and clinical phenotype can help guide genetic testing.

Autosomal Dominant Osteogenesis Imperfecta

Autosomal dominant mutations in COL1A1 or COL1A2 account for approximately 90% cases of OI (see **Table 1**).[5] Type I OI arises from a quantitative defect in collagen production due to a silenced allele of the COL1A1 gene.[6] Usually as a result of a premature stop codon within the gene,[7] these mutations lead to half of the normal amount of protein production. The structure of the type 1 collagen protein that is produced is normal. Type 1 OI presents with fractures, typically before puberty, and is nondeforming. With the completion of growth the incidence of fractures decreases.

In comparison, type II, III, and IV OI are a result of structural defects in type I collagen due to missense mutations in either the COL1A1 or COL1A2 gene. The most common mutations, involving substitution of glycine by a larger amino acid, disrupt the triple helix assembly of collagen, impairing its function and interactions with the extracellular matrix.[8] Depending on the helical location of a mutation and the resultant instability of the protein, the clinical phenotype can range from lethal to mildly deforming.

Table 1
Autosomal dominant mutations involved in osteogenesis imperfecta

Gene	Condition	Disease Mechanism	Skeletal Phenotype	Associated Features
COL1A1	OI type I	Decreased type I collagen production	Mild	Nondeforming, most fractures prepubertal, presenile deafness, aortic regurgitation
COL1A1 COL1A2	OI type II	Abnormal type 1 collagen production	Lethal	Multiple rib, long bone and vertebral fractures, pulmonary hypoplasia, central nervous system malformations and hemorrhages
	OI type III	Abnormal type 1 collagen production	Severe	Triangular facies, short stature, severe long bone deformities, elongated vertebral pedicles, "popcorn" appearance of metaphyses and epiphyses, decreased ability to ambulate
	OI type IV	Abnormal type 1 collagen production	Moderate	Short stature, may have long bone bowing, scoliosis, and joint laxity
IFITM5	OI type V	Dysregulation of collagen mineralization	Moderate	Calcification of forearm intraosseous membrane, radial head dislocation, hyperplastic callous formation

Table 2
Autosomal recessive mutations involved in osteogenesis imperfecta

Gene	Condition	Disease Mechanism	Skeletal Phenotype	Associated Features
SERPINF1	OI type VI	Mineralization defect	Moderate to severe	Healthy at birth with subsequent progressively severe deformities. Undermineralization and "fish-scale" pattern on iliac crest biopsies
CRTAP	OI type VII	Collagen 3-hydroxylation defect	Severe to lethal	Rhizomelia, neonatal fractures, popcorn metaphyses, short stature
LEPRE1	OI type VIII	Collagen 3-hydroxylation defect	Severe to lethal	Rhizomelia, popcorn metaphyses, short stature
PPIB	OI type IX	Collagen 3-hydroxylation defect	Severe	Short stature
SERPINH1	OI type X	Chaperone defect	Severe	Renal stones
FKBP10	OI type XI	Chaperone defect	Moderate to severe	Contractures
BMP1	OI type XII	Defective collagen processing	Severe	Hyperextensibility
SP7	Unclassified	Impaired osteoblast differentiation	Moderate	Delayed tooth eruption
WNT1	Unclassified	Impaired osteoblast function	Moderate to severe	Central nervous system malformations

Type II OI is the most severe form of OI and newborns do not generally survive past the perinatal period. Infants present with multiple intrauterine fractures and severe long bone deformities. Pulmonary hypoplasia with multiple rib fractures or central nervous malformations usually result in death.[9] Type III OI is the most severe, nonlethal form and is characterized by history of multiple fractures from infancy, severe long bone deformities, and significant short stature. Children have typical triangular facies from a relatively large skull with underdeveloped facial bones. Multiple vertebral compression fractures cause severe scoliosis, kyphosis, and rib cage deformity. Distortion of the growth plates with partial calcification of cartilage can lead to a popcorn appearance of epiphyses. Ambulation is often limited either to a wheelchair or with aids. Type IV OI, although not as severe as type III, can present with some long limb bowing, vertebral fractures, and relative short stature. Most children are ambulatory, although may need walking aids.

Individuals with type V OI exhibit specific clinical features including calcification of the forearm intraosseous membrane, radiodense metaphyseal bands at growth plates of long bones, and development of hyperplastic callus after trauma.[10] There is an 85% incidence of radial head dislocation.[11] Genetic mutations in the gene encoding interferon-induced transmembrane protein 5 (IFITM5) were discovered in 2012 to be the causative defect.[12] Although IFITM5 appears to play a role in bone ossification, the mechanism by which it regulates collagen mineralization is not known.[13]

Autosomal Recessive Osteogenesis Imperfecta

The autosomal recessive forms of OI are rare conditions and account for approximately 2% to 5% of cases. Mutations have been discovered in critical elements involved in type I collagen secretion and post-translation modification (collagen 3-hydroxylation and chaperone defects)[14–16] as well as signaling and transcription factors involved in osteoblast function (see **Table 2**).[17–19] Although the autosomal recessive forms are uncommon, the discovery of multiple new genes responsible for OI has shed light onto new mechanistic pathways and possible therapeutic approaches.

EXTRASKELETAL CLINICAL FEATURES OF OSTEOGENESIS IMPERFECTA
Hearing Loss

The hearing loss, a mixture of conductive and sensorineural deficiency, is generally progressive, with 50% of adults with OI having hearing loss by 50 years of age (**Box 1**).[20] The prevalence of hearing difficulties in children with OI is around 5%.[21]

Dental Abnormalities

Dentinogenesis imperfecta is characterized by abnormal dentin leading to the appearance of small deformed teeth, which are opalescent due to a higher ratio of transparent enamel to opaque dentin.[22] Primary dentition is more affected than the permanent dentition. The prevalence of dentinogenesis imperfecta in patients with OI is approximately 28%.[23] Malocclusion and delayed tooth eruption can occur in up to 60% to 80% of patients.[23]

Ocular Changes

Patients with OI frequently have blue sclera, particularly in type I OI. The scleral color can vary and is generally darker in infancy.

Box 1
Extra-skeletal manifestations of osteogenesis imperfecta

Hearing loss

Dental abnormalities

- Dentinogenesis imperfecta
- Malocclusion

Blue/grey sclera

Connective tissue features

- Joint hyperextensibility

Hypercalcuria

Cardiovascular involvement

- Aortic root dilatation

Neurological features

- Macrocephaly
- Hydrocephalus
- Basilar invagination

Connective Tissue Features

Joint hyperlaxity is common and can lead to dislocation of joints and the head of the radius.[11] Abnormalities in type I collagen can also result in increased capillary fragility and bruising, decreased elasticity of skin, and hernias.[24]

Hypercalciuria

Hypercalciuria can occur in up to 36% of patients[25] and there is an increased risk for renal calculi.[3]

Cardiovascular Features

In adults with OI, aortic root dilation followed by mitral valve prolapse is the most frequent valvular manifestation.[26,27]

Neurologic Features

Macrocephaly and hydrocephalus are associated with OI.[28] Basilar invagination (an infolding of the skull case that leads to brainstem distortion) is a rare but potentially fatal complication of OI.[29] Symptoms of basilar invagination include headache, lower cranial nerve palsies, dysphagia, quadriparesis, ataxia, and nystagmus. Early intervention with occipitocervical bracing can delay progression.[30] Cervical spine kyphosis may also rarely cause compression of the cervical spinal cord. Symptoms can include sensory or motor disturbances of the upper or lower extremities progressing to quadriparesis.

DIAGNOSIS AND DIFFERENTIAL

A diagnosis of OI is based on typical clinical and radiological findings. Radiographic features include generalized osteopenia, gracile long bones with evidence of bowing (**Fig. 2**). Vertebral fractures are common, with a 71% reported prevalence rate in type 1 OI.[31] Spiral and transverse fractures of long bones are seen most commonly in the

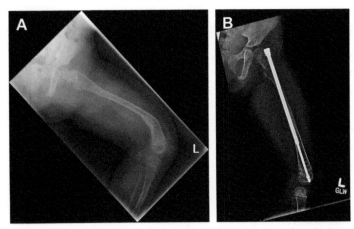

Fig. 2. (*A*) A lateral view of the femur shows thin cortices, coarse trabeculation, and deformity from a malunited fracture at the distal metadiaphyseal junction. (*B*) The same femur following osteotomy and placement of a growing intramedullary rod. Notice transverse radiodense growth lines parallel to the femoral and tibial growth plates, indicative of cyclical bisphosphonate infusion.

lower limbs,[31] and avulsion type fractures, such as olecranon and patellar fractures, occur due to decreased tensile strength of the bone (**Fig. 3**).[32] Bone mineral density as measured by dual energy radiographic absorptiometry is usually low, but is not specific or diagnostic of OI. Genetic testing can help confirm the diagnosis; however, given that more than 1500 dominant mutations in COL1A1 or COL1A2 have been identified to date, genetic sequencing of either peripheral blood or cultured fibroblasts is required. When feasible, a bone biopsy with histomorphometric analysis may provide additional diagnostic information.

In infants, nonaccidental injury (NAI) is an important diagnosis to differentiate from OI. Although the pattern of fractures (such as posterior rib and metaphyseal fractures) and associated clinical signs of injury (retinal hemorrhage, bruises) may be contributory, differentiating NAI from OI can be difficult. Although typically associated with NAI, rib fractures can be seen in up to 22% of children with OI.[33]

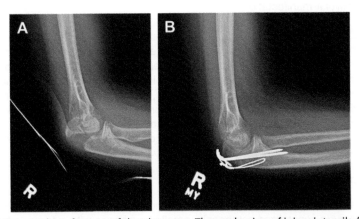

Fig. 3. (*A*) An avulsion fracture of the olecranon. The mechanism of injury is tensile failure of bone. Half of children with olecranon fractures have osteogenesis imperfecta. (*B*) Postoperative radiograph showing repair of the olecranon fracture with a tension band wiring technique.

In older children, idiopathic juvenile osteoporosis (IJO) can also present with a history of frequent fractures. Characteristically typified by bone pain and vertebral fractures before the onset of puberty, the underlying cause has yet to be identified. Transiliac histomorphometry studies in patients with IJO demonstrate decreased trabecular bone volume, number, and thickness.[34] Secondary causes of osteoporosis such as malabsorption, glucocorticoid-induced osteoporosis, hormone deficiencies, acute lymphoblastic leukemia, and immobility should be able to be differentiated based on history and laboratory investigations. Other skeletal disorders resembling OI may also need to be considered in the differential (**Table 3**).

MANAGEMENT

The goals of treatment of OI are to maximize mobility and daily life competencies and decrease bone pain and bone fragility. Management should be multidisciplinary and includes rehabilitation, surgical, and pharmacologic treatment. The degree of intervention needed depends on the severity of the clinical phenotype.[35]

Rehabilitation

Physical therapy is used to guide motor skills acquisition for severely involved children and is important in maximizing weight-bearing exercise to prevent fractures or during

Table 3
Skeletal conditions resembling osteogenesis imperfecta

Condition	Genes	Disease Mechanism	Inheritance	Associated Clinical Features
Osteoporosis pseudoglioma syndrome	LRP5	Impaired Wnt signaling and osteoblast function	AR	Congenital blindness due to vitreoretinal abnormalities
Bruck syndrome	PLOD2	Impaired collagen crosslink formation	AR	Congenital contractures
Ehlers-Danlos syndrome	COL5A1, COL5A2, TNXb, COL3A1	Connective tissue defects	AD	Joint and skin laxity, easy bruising, mitral and tricuspid prolapse
Hypophosphatasia	ALPL	Defective bone mineralization from low alkaline phosphatase activity	AD, AR	Low alkaline phosphatase
Idiopathic hyperphosphatasia	TNFRSSFIIB	Excessive bone resorption and formation	AR	Increased alkaline phosphatase, thickening of the skull vault
Idiopathic juvenile osteoporosis	Unknown	Unknown	Unknown	No extraskeletal abnormalities. Vertebral compression fractures are common

Abbreviations: AD, autosomal dominant; AR, autosomal recessive.

recovery from fractures. The heterogeneity of the patient population requires a multi-disciplinary approach to setting goals and monitoring progress. Hydrotherapy is a useful means of gradual return to weight-bearing. Wheelchairs and walking aids are prescribed according to the child's needs, with an ongoing negotiation of the balance between seated mobility for its practical use and weight-bearing exercise to maintain bone strength and ability to assist with transfers. Patients with upper extremity deformities may benefit from occupational therapy assessment to help with self-care and daily living activities.

Surgical Treatment

Fractures are the most common reason for a child with OI to see a surgeon. Fracture healing times for children with OI are normal even with bisphosphonate treatment.[36] Excessive immobilization is to be avoided during fracture treatment because it leads to weak, stiff muscles and secondary disuse osteopenia of the bones, which in turn can lead to more fractures.

Fractures in infants are best treated with the simplest form of immobilization with the aim of providing comfort to the limb while the initial fracture callus forms. Fractures heal quickly in infants (2–3 weeks). Once the limb is comfortable and stable an early return to function with guidance from a physical therapist is appropriate.

Toddlers and older children vary considerably in the number of fractures they experience and in the amount of limb deformity that occurs. Limb deformity is a combination of that resulting from healed fractures, as well as additional gradual distortion of the shape of the bone. Some children with OI have little deformity and have fracture patterns similar to those seen in the normal child population. These types of fractures are treated with closed or open management using standard techniques. Plate fixation should be avoided if possible because there is a higher risk of subsequent peri-implant fracture. There is an increased incidence of purely tensile failure of bone—for example transverse fractures of the olecranon or patella—in children with OI.[32] These respond well to tension band wiring and early motion.

Deformities of the femurs and tibiae can be treated with osteotomy and intramedullary rodding either at the time of a fracture or electively. Intramedullary rodding maintains a straight mechanical alignment and supports the whole bone, producing the best biomechanical circumstance for further strengthening with subsequent weight bearing. Modern intramedullary rods are designed to elongate as the child grows. Such growing rods have the advantage of ongoing support and a reduced number of revision operations.[37]

Scoliosis and kyphosis of the thoracolumbar spine are common in children with severe OI. Bracing is controversial particularly in younger children, because there is no evidence that it prevents the progression of scoliosis[38,39] and because there are concerns about limiting chest wall growth and contributing to restrictive lung disease. Scoliosis is not painful and does not usually interfere with sitting balance or activities of daily living. Spinal fusion with instrumentation has been reported in selected cases but has a high complication rate and is not universally recommended.[40]

Spondylolysis and spondylolisthesis of the lumbosacral spine are observed radiographically in patients with OI but are reported to occur no more frequently than in the general population.[41] This condition is usually minimally symptomatic or asymptomatic and is most often successfully managed nonoperatively.

Cervical spine abnormalities can include kyphosis or spondylolysis and spondylolisthesis. Rarely a progressive and severe cervical spine deformity will threaten or compromise cervical cord function. In these cases, careful consideration of operative decompression and fusion, with attendant high complication rates, is warranted.[42,43]

Pharmacologic Treatment

Children with OI should be assessed to ensure that there is sufficient dietary calcium and 25-hydroxyvitamin D intake. One in four children with OI has evidence of vitamin D deficiency, and serum 25-hydroxyvitamin D concentrations are independently associated with bone mineral density.[44] The decision to start pharmacotherapy, such as bisphosphonates, depends on the clinical severity of the child (presence of long bone deformities, bone pain, frequent fractures) rather than the bone mineral density or collagen mutation status.

Bisphosphonates

Bisphosphonates are analogues of pyrophosphate that bind avidly to the hydroxyapatite crystals in mineralized bone. They decrease osteoclast function and number and thereby inhibit bone resorption.[45] Transiliac histomorphometry studies have shown that intravenous bisphosphonates decrease bone resorption on endocortical surfaces while not significantly affecting osteoblast activity on periosteal surfaces, leading to increased cortical bone thickness.[46] They are the most widely used pharmacologic treatment in children with OI.

Both controlled and observational trials have demonstrated bisphosphonates significantly increase bone mineral density, with the most gain achieved within the first 2 to 4 years.[34] Although observational trials have documented reductions in long bone fracture rate and bone pain, as well as improved vertebral morphology, strength, and activities of daily living,[47–49] these results have not always been supported with results from randomized control trials. A summary of randomized controlled trial results of bisphosphonate use in children with OI is outlined in **Table 4**.[50–57]

There remain uncertainties about the optimal bisphosphonate dosing schedule and duration. Oral dosing has the advantage of convenience for patients and families but there has been concern about its effectiveness in children with more significant disease. Stopping bisphosphonate treatment while growth remains can result in a reduction in metaphyseal bone mineral content,[58] an increased risk for fracture at the junction of the untreated and treated bone.[58] However, given the decade-plus half-life of bisphosphonates in bone and concerns of the effect of continuous use on bone matrix quality[59] and potential risk for atypical fractures,[60] many clinicians have advocated for intermittent treatment. To date, there have not been any randomized controlled trials to address the optimal treatment duration.

Bisphosphonate treatment is associated with flulike symptoms in up to 85% of children following the first dose and can lead to transient hypocalcemia.[61] Decreased bone remodeling associated with treatment can delay the healing of osteotomy sites following intramedullary rodding.[62] Osteonecrosis of the jaw has been described in adult patients on bisphosphonate therapy[63] but has not reported in pediatric patients with OI to date.

Growth hormone

Growth hormone has been trialed given its potential anabolic effects on bone through stimulation of osteoblasts, collagen synthesis, and bone growth.[64] Growth hormone deficiency is uncommon in children with OI.[65] Growth hormone treatment can however increase growth velocity in children with OI,[66,67] although there are no data on its effect on final adult height. Growth hormone has been shown to increase

Table 4
Randomized controlled trials of bisphosphonate use in children with osteogenesis imperfecta

				Effect of Intervention		
Study	Intervention	Subjects	Peripheral Fracture Rate	Vertebral Fracture Rate	Lumbar Spine BMD	Bone Pain
Oral bisphosphonate randomized trials						
Sakkers et al,[50] 2004	Olpadronate vs placebo for 2 y	n = 34 10.4 ± 3.5 y (range 3–18)	31% decrease	No difference	Increased (gain of 1.67 SD vs 0.14 SD)	n/a
Seikaly et al,[51] 2005	Alendronate vs placebo for 1 y	n = 20 9.8 ± 1.1 y (range 3–15)	No difference	No difference	Increased (gain of 0.89 SD vs loss of 0.12 SD)	Decreased
Ward et al,[52] 2011	Alendronate vs placebo for 2 y	n = 139 11 ± 3.7 y (range 4–18)	No difference	No difference	Increased (gain of 1.32 SD vs 0.14 SD)	No difference
Bishop et al,[53] 2013	Risedronate vs placebo for 1 y	n = 143 8.8 ± 3.4 y (range 4–15)	47% decrease	No difference	Increased (gain of 16.3% vs 7.6%)	No difference
Intravenous bisphosphonate randomized trials						
Letocha et al,[54] 2005	Pamidronate vs no treatment for 1 y	n = 18 11.1 ± 2.4 y (range 7–13)	Decreased upper but not lower extremity fractures	Increased vertebral height	Increased (gain of 1.4 SD vs no change)	No difference
Gatti et al,[55] 2005	Neridronate vs no treatment for 1 y	n = 66 8.7 ± 2.3 y (range 6–11)	No difference in percentage of subjects with fractures, 64% reduction in total number of fractures	Increased vertebral area	Increased (gain of 18%–25% vs 3.5%–5.7%)	n/a
Bisphosphonate comparison randomized trials						
DiMeglio et al,[56] 2006	Alendronate vs pamidronate for 2 y	n = 18 8.7 y (range 3–17)	No difference between groups	n/a	No difference between groups (gain of 2.1 SD vs 1.9 SD)	n/a
Barros et al,[57] 2012	Pamidronate vs zoledronic acid	n = 23 7.6 ± 4.5 y (range 1–16)	Decrease in fracture rate in both groups compared with baseline with no difference between groups	n/a	Greater gain in zoledronic acid group (gain of 2.5 SD vs 1.5 SD)	n/a

Abbreviations: BMD, bone mineral density as measured by dual energy radiographic absorptiometry; n/a, not assessed; SD, standard deviation.

bone mineral density either alone[66] or in combination with bisphosphonate treatment[67] but has not been demonstrated to decrease fracture rate. Currently there is insufficient evidence to support the standard use of growth hormone in children with OI.

Potential future therapies
Receptor activator of nuclear factor-κB ligand inhibitors, such as denosumab, inhibit osteoclast formation and bone degradation. In a mouse model of OI, denosumab increased bone density and cortical thickness and decreased fracture rate.[68] There has been one study in 4 children with type VI OI, which demonstrated denosumab normalized previously elevated markers of bone resorption.[69] Further data of its effect on fracture rate and bone pain in children with OI are still needed.

Antisclerostin and Dickkopf-1 antibodies increase osteoblast activity and periosteal bone formation through inhibition of the Wnt pathway.[70] Sclerostin antibody treatment in mice models of OI have shown improvement in long bone fragility[71] and may offer a potential new therapy option for children with OI in the future.

The current pharmacologic agents do not correct the primary underlying cause of OI. There is ongoing work looking at gene and molecular therapy options. Approaches in animal models that have been trialed include down-regulating the expression of the defective collagen allele through short interfering RNAs or ribozymes.[72] Infusions of mesenchymal stem cells with osteoblast potential have lead to improvements in bone phenotypes in mice models of OI.[73] Minimal benefits, however, were seen in a small group of children with severe OI who were given a bone marrow transplant indicating much more research is still needed in this area before clinical application.[74]

SUMMARY

The last 10 years have led to substantial advances in the understanding of underlying mechanisms, genetics, and potential treatment options for children with OI. Management involves a multidisciplinary approach with rehabilitation, surgical management, and consideration of bisphosphonate therapy. Further research is still needed to clarify uncertainties around treatment duration and schedule, as well as to explore alternative more targeted therapeutic modalities.

REFERENCES

1. Stevenson DA, Carey JC, Byrne JL, et al. Analysis of skeletal dysplasias in the utah population. Am J Med Genet A 2012;158A(5):1046–54.
2. Stoll C, Dott B, Roth MP, et al. Birth prevalence rates of skeletal dysplasias. Clin Genet 1989;35(2):88–92.
3. Vetter U, Pontz B, Zauner E, et al. Osteogenesis imperfecta: a clinical study of the first ten years of life. Calcif Tissue Int 1992;50(1):36–41.
4. Sillence DO, Senn A, Danks DM. Genetic heterogeneity in osteogenesis imperfecta. J Med Genet 1979;16(2):101–16.
5. Bodian DL, Chan TF, Poon A, et al. Mutation and polymorphism spectrum in osteogenesis imperfecta type II: implications for genotype-phenotype relationships. Hum Mol Genet 2009;18(3):463–71.
6. Willing MC, Deschenes SP, Scott DA, et al. Osteogenesis imperfecta type I: molecular heterogeneity for COL1A1 null alleles of type I collagen. Am J Hum Genet 1994;55(4):638–47.

7. Slayton RL, Deschenes SP, Willing MC. Nonsense mutations in the COL1A1 gene preferentially reduce nuclear levels of mRNA but not hnRNA in osteogenesis imperfecta type I cell strains. Matrix Biol 2000;19(1):1–9.

8. Marini JC, Forlino A, Cabral WA, et al. Consortium for osteogenesis imperfecta mutations in the helical domain of type I collagen: regions rich in lethal mutations align with collagen binding sites for integrins and proteoglycans. Hum Mutat 2007;28(3):209–21.

9. McAllion SJ, Paterson CR. Causes of death in osteogenesis imperfecta. J Clin Pathol 1996;49(8):627–30.

10. Glorieux FH, Rauch F, Plotkin H, et al. Type V osteogenesis imperfecta: a new form of brittle bone disease. J Bone Miner Res 2000;15(9):1650–8.

11. Fassier AM, Rauch F, Aarabi M, et al. Radial head dislocation and subluxation in osteogenesis imperfecta. J Bone Joint Surg Am 2007;89(12):2694–704.

12. Semler O, Garbes L, Keupp K, et al. A mutation in the 5'-UTR of IFITM5 creates an in-frame start codon and causes autosomal-dominant osteogenesis imperfecta type V with hyperplastic callus. Am J Hum Genet 2012;91(2):349–57.

13. Marini JC, Blissett AR. New genes in bone development: what's new in osteogenesis imperfecta. J Clin Endocrinol Metab 2013;98(8):3095–103.

14. Becker J, Semler O, Gilissen C, et al. Exome sequencing identifies truncating mutations in human SERPINF1 in autosomal-recessive osteogenesis imperfecta. Am J Hum Genet 2011;88(3):362–71.

15. Barnes AM, Carter EM, Cabral WA, et al. Lack of cyclophilin B in osteogenesis imperfecta with normal collagen folding. N Engl J Med 2010;362(6):521–8.

16. Alanay Y, Avaygan H, Camacho N, et al. Mutations in the gene encoding the RER protein FKBP65 cause autosomal-recessive osteogenesis imperfecta. Am J Hum Genet 2010;86(4):551–9.

17. Martinez-Glez V, Valencia M, Caparros-Martin JA, et al. Identification of a mutation causing deficient BMP1/mTLD proteolytic activity in autosomal recessive osteogenesis imperfecta. Hum Mutat 2012;33(2):343–50.

18. Lapunzina P, Aglan M, Temtamy S, et al. Identification of a frameshift mutation in osterix in a patient with recessive osteogenesis imperfecta. Am J Hum Genet 2010;87(1):110–4.

19. Laine CM, Joeng KS, Campeau PM, et al. WNT1 mutations in early-onset osteoporosis and osteogenesis imperfecta. N Engl J Med 2013;368(19):1809–16.

20. Paterson CR, Monk EA, McAllion SJ. How common is hearing impairment in osteogenesis imperfecta? J Laryngol Otol 2001;115(4):280–2.

21. Kuurila K, Grenman R, Johansson R, et al. Hearing loss in children with osteogenesis imperfecta. Eur J Pediatr 2000;159(7):515–9.

22. Majorana A, Bardellini E, Brunelli PC, et al. Dentinogenesis imperfecta in children with osteogenesis imperfecta: a clinical and ultrastructural study. Int J Paediatr Dent 2010;20(2):112–8.

23. O'Connell AC, Marini JC. Evaluation of oral problems in an osteogenesis imperfecta population. Oral Surg Oral Med Oral Pathol Oral Radiol Endod 1999;87(2):189–96.

24. Hansen B, Jemec GB. The mechanical properties of skin in osteogenesis imperfecta. Arch Dermatol 2002;138(7):909–11.

25. Chines A, Boniface A, McAlister W, et al. Hypercalciuria in osteogenesis imperfecta: a follow-up study to assess renal effects. Bone 1995;16(3):333–9.

26. Bonita RE, Cohen IS, Berko BA. Valvular heart disease in osteogenesis imperfecta: presentation of a case and review of the literature. Echocardiography 2010;27(1):69–73.

27. White NJ, Winearls CG, Smith R. Cardiovascular abnormalities in osteogenesis imperfecta. Am Heart J 1983;106(6):1416–20.
28. Charnas LR, Marini JC. Communicating hydrocephalus, basilar invagination, and other neurologic features in osteogenesis imperfecta. Neurology 1993; 43(12):2603–8.
29. Forlino A, Cabral WA, Barnes AM, et al. New perspectives on osteogenesis imperfecta. Nat Rev Endocrinol 2011;7(9):540–57.
30. Menezes AH. Specific entities affecting the craniocervical region: osteogenesis imperfecta and related osteochondrodysplasias: Medical and surgical management of basilar impression. Childs Nerv Syst 2008;24(10):1169–72.
31. Ben Amor IM, Roughley P, Glorieux FH, et al. Skeletal clinical characteristics of osteogenesis imperfecta caused by haploinsufficiency mutations in COL1A1. J Bone Miner Res 2013;28(9):2001–7.
32. Stott NS, Zionts LE. Displaced fractures of the apophysis of the olecranon in children who have osteogenesis imperfecta. J Bone Joint Surg Am 1993; 75(7):1026–33.
33. Greeley CS, Donaruma-Kwoh M, Vettimattam M, et al. Fractures at diagnosis in infants and children with osteogenesis imperfecta. J Pediatr Orthop 2013;33(1): 32–6.
34. Rauch F, Plotkin H, Zeitlin L, et al. Bone mass, size, and density in children and adolescents with osteogenesis imperfecta: effect of intravenous pamidronate therapy. J Bone Miner Res 2003;18(4):610–4.
35. Engelbert RH, Uiterwaal CS, Gerver WJ, et al. Osteogenesis imperfecta in childhood: Impairment and disability. A prospective study with 4-year follow-up. Arch Phys Med Rehabil 2004;85(5):772–8.
36. Pizones J, Plotkin H, Parra-Garcia JI, et al. Bone healing in children with osteogenesis imperfecta treated with bisphosphonates. J Pediatr Orthop 2005;25(3):332–5.
37. Fassier F, Glorieux FH. Surgical management of osteogenesis imperfecta. In: Duparc J, editor. Surgical techniques in orthopaedics and traumatology. Paris: Elsevier SAS; 2003. p. 1–8.
38. Yong-Hing K, MacEwen GD. Scoliosis associated with osteogenesis imperfecta. J Bone Joint Surg Br 1982;64(1):36–43.
39. Benson DR, Donaldson DH, Millar EA. The spine in osteogenesis imperfecta. J Bone Joint Surg Am 1978;60(7):925–9.
40. Topouchian V, Finidori G, Glorion C, et al. Posterior spinal fusion for kyphoscoliosis associated with osteogenesis imperfecta: long-term results. Rev Chir Orthop Reparatrice Appar Mot 2004;90(6):525–32.
41. Verra WC, Pruijs HJ, Beek EJ, et al. Prevalence of vertebral pars defects (spondylolysis) in a population with osteogenesis imperfecta. Spine (Phila Pa 1976) 2009;34(13):1399–401.
42. Daivajna S, Jones A, Hossein Mehdian SM. Surgical management of severe cervical kyphosis with myelopathy in osteogenesis imperfecta: a case report. Spine (Phila Pa 1976) 2005;30(7):E191–4.
43. Sasaki-Adams D, Kulkarni A, Rutka J, et al. Neurosurgical implications of osteogenesis imperfecta in children. report of 4 cases. J Neurosurg Pediatr 2008; 1(3):229–36.
44. Edouard T, Glorieux FH, Rauch F. Relationship between vitamin D status and bone mineralization, mass, and metabolism in children with osteogenesis imperfecta: histomorphometric study. J Bone Miner Res 2011;26(9):2245–51.
45. Russell RG. Bisphosphonates: mode of action and pharmacology. Pediatrics 2007;119(Suppl 2):S150–62.

46. Rauch F, Travers R, Plotkin H, et al. The effects of intravenous pamidronate on the bone tissue of children and adolescents with osteogenesis imperfecta. J Clin Invest 2002;110(9):1293–9.

47. Glorieux FH, Bishop NJ, Plotkin H, et al. Cyclic administration of pamidronate in children with severe osteogenesis imperfecta. N Engl J Med 1998;339(14): 947–52.

48. Land C, Rauch F, Munns CF, et al. Vertebral morphometry in children and adolescents with osteogenesis imperfecta: effect of intravenous pamidronate treatment. Bone 2006;39(4):901–6.

49. Lowing K, Astrom E, Oscarsson KA, et al. Effect of intravenous pamidronate therapy on everyday activities in children with osteogenesis imperfecta. Acta Paediatr 2007;96(8):1180–3.

50. Sakkers R, Kok D, Engelbert R, et al. Skeletal effects and functional outcome with olpadronate in children with osteogenesis imperfecta: a 2-year randomised placebo-controlled study. Lancet 2004;363(9419):1427–31.

51. Seikaly MG, Kopanati S, Salhab N, et al. Impact of alendronate on quality of life in children with osteogenesis imperfecta. J Pediatr Orthop 2005;25(6): 786–91.

52. Ward LM, Rauch F, Whyte MP, et al. Alendronate for the treatment of pediatric osteogenesis imperfecta: a randomized placebo-controlled study. J Clin Endocrinol Metab 2011;96(2):355–64.

53. Bishop N, Adami S, Ahmed SF, et al. Risedronate in children with osteogenesis imperfecta: a randomised, double-blind, placebo-controlled trial. Lancet 2013; 382(9902):1424–32.

54. Letocha AD, Cintas HL, Troendle JF, et al. Controlled trial of pamidronate in children with types III and IV osteogenesis imperfecta confirms vertebral gains but not short-term functional improvement. J Bone Miner Res 2005;20(6):977–86.

55. Gatti D, Antoniazzi F, Prizzi R, et al. Intravenous neridronate in children with osteogenesis imperfecta: a randomized controlled study. J Bone Miner Res 2005;20(5):758–63.

56. DiMeglio LA, Peacock M. Two-year clinical trial of oral alendronate versus intravenous pamidronate in children with osteogenesis imperfecta. J Bone Miner Res 2006;21(1):132–40.

57. Barros ER, Saraiva GL, de Oliveira TP, et al. Safety and efficacy of a 1-year treatment with zoledronic acid compared with pamidronate in children with osteogenesis imperfecta. J Pediatr Clin Endocrinol Metab 2012;25(5–6):485–91.

58. Rauch F, Munns C, Land C, et al. Pamidronate in children and adolescents with osteogenesis imperfecta: effect of treatment discontinuation. J Pediatr Clin Endocrinol Metab 2006;91(4):1268–74.

59. Kashii M, Hashimoto J, Nakano T, et al. Alendronate treatment promotes bone formation with a less anisotropic microstructure during intramembranous ossification in rats. J Bone Miner Metab 2008;26(1):24–33.

60. Nicolaou N, Agrawal Y, Padman M, et al. Changing pattern of femoral fractures in osteogenesis imperfecta with prolonged use of bisphosphonates. J Child Orthop 2012;6(1):21–7.

61. Munns CF, Rajab MH, Hong J, et al. Acute phase response and mineral status following low dose intravenous zoledronic acid in children. Bone 2007;41(3): 366–70.

62. Munns CF, Rauch F, Zeitlin L, et al. Delayed osteotomy but not fracture healing in pediatric osteogenesis imperfecta patients receiving pamidronate. J Bone Miner Res 2004;19(11):1779–86.

63. Migliorati CA, Siegel MA, Elting LS. Bisphosphonate-associated osteonecrosis: a long-term complication of bisphosphonate treatment. Lancet Oncol 2006;7(6): 508–14.

64. Giustina A, Barkan A, Chanson P, et al. Guidelines for the treatment of growth hormone excess and growth hormone deficiency in adults. J Endocrinol Invest 2008;31(9):820–38.

65. Marini JC, Bordenick S, Heavner G, et al. Evaluation of growth hormone axis and responsiveness to growth stimulation of short children with osteogenesis imperfecta. Am J Med Genet 1993;45(2):261–4.

66. Antoniazzi F, Bertoldo F, Mottes M, et al. Growth hormone treatment in osteogenesis imperfecta with quantitative defect of type I collagen synthesis. J Pediatr 1996;129(3):432–9.

67. Antoniazzi F, Monti E, Venturi G, et al. GH in combination with bisphosphonate treatment in osteogenesis imperfecta. Eur J Endocrinol 2010;163(3):479–87.

68. Bargman R, Posham R, Boskey AL, et al. Comparable outcomes in fracture reduction and bone properties with RANKL inhibition and alendronate treatment in a mouse model of osteogenesis imperfecta. Osteoporos Int 2012;23(3): 1141–50.

69. Semler O, Netzer C, Hoyer-Kuhn H, et al. First use of the RANKL antibody denosumab in osteogenesis imperfecta type VI. J Musculoskelet Neuronal Interact 2012;12(3):183–8.

70. Ke HZ, Richards WG, Li X, et al. Sclerostin and dickkopf-1 as therapeutic targets in bone diseases. Endocr Rev 2012;33(5):747–83.

71. Sinder BP, Eddy MM, Ominsky MS, et al. Sclerostin antibody improves skeletal parameters in a brtl/+ mouse model of osteogenesis imperfecta. J Bone Miner Res 2013;28(1):73–80.

72. Dawson PA, Marini JC. Hammerhead ribozymes selectively suppress mutant type I collagen mRNA in osteogenesis imperfecta fibroblasts. Nucleic Acids Res 2000;28(20):4013–20.

73. Mehrotra M, Rosol M, Ogawa M, et al. Amelioration of a mouse model of osteogenesis imperfecta with hematopoietic stem cell transplantation: microcomputed tomography studies. Exp Hematol 2010;38(7):593–602.

74. Horwitz EM, Prockop DJ, Fitzpatrick LA, et al. Transplantability and therapeutic effects of bone marrow-derived mesenchymal cells in children with osteogenesis imperfecta. Nat Med 1999;5(3):309–13.

Index

Note: Page numbers of article titles are in **boldface** type.

Pediatr Clin N Am 61 (2014) 1259–1267
http://dx.doi.org/10.1016/S0031-3955(14)00207-7
0031-3955/14/$ – see front matter © 2014 Elsevier Inc. All rights reserved.

pediatric.theclinics.com

Moving?

Make sure your subscription moves with you!

To notify us of your new address, find your **Clinics Account Number** (located on your mailing label above your name), and contact customer service at:

Email: journalscustomerservice-usa@elsevier.com

800-654-2452 (subscribers in the U.S. & Canada)
314-447-8871 (subscribers outside of the U.S. & Canada)

Fax number: 314-447-8029

**Elsevier Health Sciences Division
Subscription Customer Service
3251 Riverport Lane
Maryland Heights, MO 63043**

*To ensure uninterrupted delivery of your subscription, please notify us at least 4 weeks in advance of move.

Printed and bound by CPI Group (UK) Ltd, Croydon, CR0 4YY

03/10/2024

01040490-0017